November 2021

Thank you For reading

Lylee

Saved by a Stranger

Saved
by a
Stranger

Life-changing Journeys of
Transplant Patients

LEZLEE PETERZELL-BELLANICH

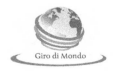

Giro di Mondo

CONTENTS

DEDICATION

This book is dedicated to all those who made the choice to donate their organs, the doctors and professionals in the transplant field making it happen, and those patients and families desperately waiting for their miracle of transplantation. Hopefully, many more people will get their second chance at life as we did.

Preface

This book not only tells our personal journey towards my husband's life-saving liver transplant, but also the remarkable survival stories of other transplant patients we have had the privilege of meeting through the Mayo Clinic's Second Chance Support Group. Just as hearing their stories helped alleviate our fears, I am hoping this book will do the same for others who are going through the transplant tunnel.

With transplant, there is hope—hope that, like a machine with a new engine part, a body can be restored. Without donors, transplant is not an option. Therefore, I hope the book will also combat myths, fears, and apathy regarding organ donation.

The national organ registry, Donate Life America, reports that more than 700,000 organ transplants, including kidney, liver, heart, and pancreas, have been performed in the United States since 1988. Yet, according to the American Transplant Foundation, liver and kidney diseases kill more than 120,000 Americans each year—more than Alzheimer's, breast cancer, or prostate cancer.

In the United States, a person must opt-in to be an organ donor by indicating consent on their driver's license or registering with a state or national registry. But there is simply too much demand

and not enough supply, so an average of twenty people die each day waiting for an organ.

Not everyone is comfortable talking about the subject because of fears surrounding unexpected death or misconceptions about the process. But these conversations, and an understanding of the organ donation system, are vital to increasing our donor population. Organ donation is the last and greatest gift imaginable.

A healthy person may decide to become a living donor and, if matched with a recipient and approved, may donate one of their kidneys or a portion of their liver— the only organ in the human body that can regenerate to its normal size.

I interviewed dozens of people for this book including pre- and post-transplant patients, living donors, doctors, and transplant professionals. Their stories and knowledge were crucial to our strength in getting through Rob's transplant.

Being sick is being vulnerable. Finding the best possible care facility, being willing to go anywhere and do anything to increase the chances of prolonged life while navigating the health insurance system, is worth the fight. Being accepted into a top-rated transplant program as we did at Mayo Clinic involves an intense educational process for both the patient and caregiver. In return, patients receive clear communication from their medical team. Good care before, during, and after a transplant breeds trust and confidence.

Having a support group of people who have undergone the same experience is invaluable. No one understands the highs, lows, anxiety, and physical and emotional transformation like these patients and caregivers. I am amazed by the entire journey of transplantation. Each of us is a powerful story.

Stories after stories. But life breaks down to one story at a time.

CHAPTER 1
The Final Anticipated Moment

September 10, 2020, St. Augustine, Florida

"How quickly can you get to the hospital?" asked Inga, the on-call Procurement nurse at Mayo Clinic.

It was a little after midnight. We had been resting in our rented condo when the phone rang, and Rob put the caller on speakerphone.

We both sat up in disbelief. "We can be there in forty-five minutes."

"Good. The liver is going to you. This is a good liver. There are no high risks. Go straight to the ER and you will be directed from there."

OMG. OMG. I grabbed a bag, stuffed some clothes in it, snatched my computer, and told our sleepy daughter, Skye, what was happening. She shot up in bed. "What? Daddy is getting a liver?"

"We don't know for sure, but we have to go to the hospital." At eleven years old, Skye fully understood the importance of this moment.

The hospital had called about a half-hour earlier to let us know there were two livers available for transplants, and one of the intended recipients might not match the size of the organ, so there was a chance Rob might be chosen instead. But we had been through this before, and it hadn't worked out.

At 12:15 a.m. Rob and I got in the car, with the Florida sky flashing lightning bolts and the rain pouring down. Wouldn't it be ironic, I thought, if we got in a car accident on the way to the hospital? As we drove to Jacksonville, I kept thinking of the donor and prayed for his or her family. Part of me felt guilty for being so grateful, knowing someone's life needed to end for Rob to receive his gift.

Rob and I both decided we did not want to tell our inner circle of people what was happening yet, in case it was another "dry run" (when the surgery appears imminent but has to be canceled). Perhaps we jinxed it last time. Still, we texted three individuals for specific reasons. Heidi, our neighbor, so she would know to take care of Skye the next morning; Andy, Rob's liver transplant support group mentor; and Jerry, another transplant recipient, both of whom had become like comrades. That was it. For the first time in my life, I kept something to myself without sharing it with family and close friends. It was real and just between us.

At 12:58 a.m. we reached the ER, checked in, and followed a nurse up to room 317. Rob went through the same prep as he had done before except this time, the anesthesiologist, Ryan, came in to talk to us, and then we met with the surgeon, Dr. Shennen Mao, a young woman in her mid-thirties. Dr. Mao was calming, with long, light brown hair, graceful, thin arms, and delicate hands.

She showed us a picture on her phone of the new donor liver, which looked pink and beautiful—both lobes. I asked Dr. Mao where she studied, and she said she went to Harvard Medical School and then Mayo Clinic in Rochester, Minnesota. "Ah, Harvard," I commented approvingly. "Rob, how do you feel about that?" He nodded in agreement.

"I have a request," Rob said to the doctor. "Can you please take a picture of my old liver and of the new liver going in?"

"Absolutely," Dr. Mao said.

A few hours passed, and at 4:15 a.m., nurses came in with a wheelchair.

"What is your name and date of birth?" one of the medical team members asked Rob, and he answered.

"And what are we doing today?"

"Liver transplant!" Rob proudly responded.

Finally, it was all coming together.

We had been waiting for more than two years—first in New York and then, since October 2019, on a waitlist in northeast Florida—for this miraculous moment. And it had been many more years of pain, stress, tension, and worry since Rob was diagnosed with a progressive illness that had no known cause and could not be cured without a transplant.

Now, while my husband went to the operating room, there would be more waiting for me during the surgery. I had time to reflect on how much had happened in our lives, what we'd gone through, and everyone who had been part of our journey.

CHAPTER 2

A Captain Meets a Singer/Songwriter

August 1999, New York City

I met my husband, Rob Bellanich, simply by chance while visiting a college friend, Roger, whom I had not seen in ten years. At the time, I was a singer/songwriter living in my one-bedroom apartment on the Upper West Side of Manhattan. It's hard to remember life before cell phones or social media, but somehow, my friend tracked me down and invited me to a small gathering onboard his catamaran sailing vessel at the Lincoln Harbor Yacht Club marina across the Hudson River.

Having just finished a three-week tour playing venues throughout Germany, I was feeling upbeat on that clear sunny day. Carrying my guitar inside my backpack case, I boarded a NY Waterway ferry across to Weehawken, New Jersey. Roger met me at the marina entrance, and I trailed behind him down the dock. Suddenly, an enthusiastic man with a distinct New Jersey accent called out to me from the stern of his Chris Craft motor yacht with the intriguing name *Risk it All*. Growing up in Atlanta, with a slight Southern drawl, I was particularly aware of regional dialects.

"Hey, where are ya goin'?" he asked.

"I'm heading to Roger's boat," I answered.

"Yeah, I'll be there soon to help him cruise out to da Statue."

Once on my friend's boat, I realized I needed a hat for shade. He

14

didn't have one but suggested I ask Captain Rob, who lived three boats down. So I walked back down the dock and, without permission, entered *Risk it All,* only to discover the man I'd just spoken to was coming out of the shower with a towel wrapped around his waist. I'm not going to lie. I couldn't help but notice that he had a nice, manly-looking chest. Embarrassed, I apologized while he laughed and smoothed his hair back with his hands. That was the beginning of our easy friendship, which quickly developed into an unexpected romance.

Within the close-knit, live-aboard boating community, Rob was affectionately known as "Captain Rob," a title he was proud of. He was also known as the "go-to" guy who would happily help anyone with a boating question. Encouraged by a man named Captain Nat who was like his "dock dad," he had recently obtained his 100-ton captain's license and began chartering his vessel for up to six passengers. Captain Rob took guests around lower Manhattan for private gatherings, marriage proposals, and photo shoots cruising right in the front of the Statue of Liberty.

On paper, Rob and I were very different. In fact, I had never met anyone quite like him, but there was something pure and honest about this captain that appealed to me. His Italian mother, Rosanna, met her husband, Antonio "Nino," in Italy after he left the tiny Croatian island called Illovic to become a merchant marine. Rosanna and Nino, who spoke both Croatian and Italian, came to the United States in 1962 and raised their four sons, Marco, Giampaolo, Robert and Stephen in Union City, New Jersey, also known as "Little Cuba." Therefore, Rob and his brothers spoke Italian in the home, Spanish on the streets, and English in the classroom.

My parents, Becky Hoffman and Marc Peterzell, raised me in the suburbs of Atlanta, Georgia. Originally from Mobile, Alabama, my mother earned a bachelor's and a master's degree, and my father was a law school graduate. After a few years in Manhattan, they moved to Atlanta where my father practiced as an attorney for forty-nine years at the same firm, Arnall Golden Gregory. Mom was a teacher, drummer, and after her divorce, a world traveler and licensed tour guide.

Brought up Catholic, Rob had two Jewish ex-wives, so he was initially spooked that I, too, was Jewish, even though religion was not a big part of either of our lives. Knowing I was a struggling artist, he paid double for my latest studio album and asked if I would help him as a first mate on his charters.

I liked handling the lines, had fun watching people enjoying themselves afloat, and marveled at how Rob could fix just about anything. He kept his comfortable vessel in immaculate condition, just as when he served in the Navy.

Listening to my recordings, he thought I was talented and arranged a dock performance, where I played on the stern of his boat while he went around the marina selling my CDs. During most of my twenties, I was dating dreamer musicians. Rob was more rooted in earthly endeavors. We got a kick out of each other. He accepted my quirkiness, and I was impressed by his innate talents. It felt right.

A year later, Rob met me in Europe on my second tour and, overcoming stage fright, proposed onstage at the Hard Rock Cafe in Prague after I sang my original song, "Risk it All," for him. After the show, I remember walking together along the cobblestone streets beneath an umbrella, feeling the delicate diamond ring on my finger and thinking, "Now we are a team." We were married August 3, 2001, aboard a lovely dinner yacht in New York Harbor.

Five weeks later, Rob was at the marina in New Jersey with a perfect view of the Twin Towers collapsing in lower Manhattan on September 11. After the Coast Guard put out a plea to all surrounding boats, a manager of a neighboring 550-passenger dinner yacht was trying to find an available captain to take the vessel across the river and rescue people from the disaster. Even though Rob had never captained a yacht that large before, he immediately volunteered and safely brought the ship across the river despite a mechanical problem.

I realized, as I would many times in the future, how amazingly calm, strong, and decisive my husband was in an emergency.

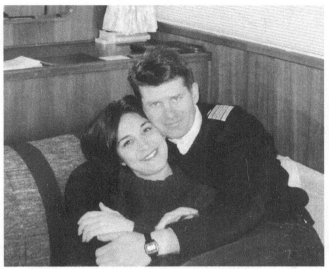

Lezlee and Rob in the fall of 1999

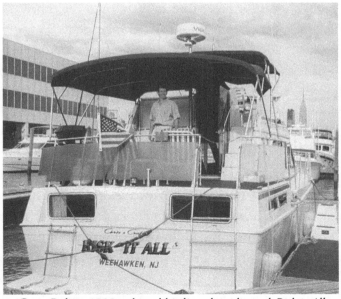

Capt. Rob in 1999 onboard his live-aboard vessel *Risk it All*

CHAPTER 3

A Shocking Diagnosis

Summer 2002, New York City

Taking my marriage vows seriously, I felt the urge to build a secure future together by combining our strengths. Rob was the visionary, and I was the implementer. With the internet beginning to explode, Rob taught himself how to build a website, and soon we were immersed in growing two businesses—one as brokerage sales event planners for other dinner yachts and the other as owner/operators of our own newly purchased dinner yacht.

We also decided to apply for life insurance, requiring simple blood tests. My test came back normal, but Rob's liver enzymes were elevated, and the insurance company declined him. As a Navy veteran, Rob had full medical coverage at any VA hospital. After his report, doctors performed a liver biopsy. They could not initially come up with a diagnosis, so we fought for and received limited life insurance coverage.

Only six months later, Rob began to develop severe gastrointestinal problems. He became weak and dehydrated from constant diarrhea. A young VA doctor diagnosed him with ulcerative colitis (UC) and put him on prescription drugs to halt the diarrhea and control the UC.

After his symptoms were controlled, the doctor ordered an MRI of his liver to see if Rob might have a rare autoimmune disease called primary sclerosing cholangitis (PSC), which also affects some people who have UC. More common in men than women, PSC is a long-term progressive autoimmune disease characterized by inflammation and scarring of the ducts in the liver that normally allow bile to drain from the gallbladder. Over time, the strictures cause buildup of bile leading to cirrhosis of the liver.

In 2003, at thirty-nine years old, Rob was officially diagnosed with PSC, only two years after we were married. According to everything we read, a liver transplant would be necessary, usually between ten and fifteen years later. We were in disbelief.

Doctors prescribed a drug to slow down the progression of PSC and then encouraged us to live our lives. Immediately, I obtained a small business health insurance plan and put Rob on it to avoid the current "preexisting condition" law so that we would have other options one day when he needed a transplant.

Getting this news at such a young age felt as if a bomb had gone off. *Boom*! It changed everything. We were shocked and scared. Should we have a child? How much time before symptoms would occur? Ironically, Rob's father had died of cirrhosis of the liver in 1981 before liver transplants were common. Could he have had PSC, and could this disease be hereditary?

Immediately after hearing this news, Rob began questioning his mortality. While he still looked and felt healthy, his mindset completely shifted. Looking back, the diagnosis itself changed him psychologically before his serious physical symptoms occurred.

Before this shock, he had been a relaxed, hard-working, passionate, extremely neat, self-employed guy who enjoyed living on his boat. He used to tell me that he believed stress was the number one cause of health problems. But after our marriage, we had "risked it all" by purchasing a 149-passenger dinner boat named *Festiva* and entering a stressful industry where one mistake could cost tens of thousands of dollars or even lives.

Thinking he had less time meant trying to fit everything in

quickly. Rob became more irritable, angry, impatient, tired, and we became less and less physically and emotionally intimate. Perhaps he was trying to psychologically protect me from getting too close, but I continually felt hurt and rejected while trying hard to live up to his expectations. Fear of death has a powerful effect on the psyche.

Rob had twin daughters from his first marriage, when he served in the Navy, but he had not seen them in many years. While that separation from his daughters had seemed an initial red flag to me, I trusted my gut, which told me he would be a good father once he was more settled in life. I also knew there are always two sides to every story.

In 2004, our business was doing well enough, and we thought it was the right time to have a child together. Our son, River, was born in 2005, a joyous time for both of us; it felt wonderful being a family. We were living in the New York City apartment where I'd lived for many years. A year after River was born, we purchased our home in Upper Nyack, New York, and Rob began renovating it voraciously.

At the end of 2007, we bought a larger yacht, *Royal Princess*, which could hold up to 180 guests. This put even more pressure on us. We were hosting private events such as weddings, corporate events, and bar/bat mitzvahs with chefs, crew, entertainment, and wait staff. Then in 2009, miraculously when I was forty-one, our daughter, Skye, was born.

Our business was all-encompassing, both mentally and physically. Even when we sold the smaller yacht to solely run the larger vessel, one wrong move could have been disastrous, but we were a good team.

As time went on, Rob's behavior became more erratic, stubborn, and impulsive. A Virgo perfectionist, he put so much pressure on himself and was often distracted by focusing on work. How much of it was caused by his disease is unclear, but I believe it affected his decision making and his ability to relax and be in the moment.

Needing answers, I joined an online PSC and UC support group.

While everyone is different, I learned that some of Rob's behavior was indeed tied to his disease. Caregivers have their own journey. Disconnecting emotionally is an important self-protective armor when your partner is ill. While my nature is upbeat, I was withering inside, which made me hate his disease even more. Like many men, Rob didn't want to talk about it. It was easier to keep busy and discuss other more pressing things.

Being more of a private person, Rob was often upset with my over-sharing. But as an artist and extrovert, I needed to get my feelings out there through music, writing, or talking. I would spend hours writing him long emails that would go unanswered or have lengthy telephone conversations with my closest friend, Mindy, because we had always shared everything since high school. And thank God for my mother, whom I could call at any time for support.

Deep down, I knew that Rob and I were good together, and if I was sick, he would be by my side every step of the way. I knew he loved me even if he had a hard time saying or showing it. I kept telling myself that I needed to hold on. Wasn't I supposed to love him in sickness and in health? That's what I believed. But, damn, we got thrown a curve ball that became a shadow over our lives.

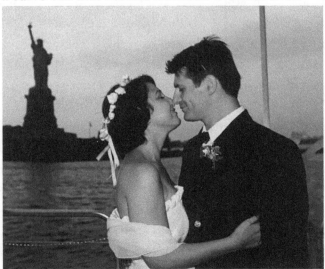

Lezlee and Rob's wedding day, August 3, 2001

CHAPTER 4

Growth Comes from Loss and Struggle

August 2019, New York

Timing in life is everything. Only a few months earlier, my beloved mother had passed away on May 4, which was also her seventy-eighth birthday. After surviving breast cancer in her forties, she was diagnosed with a rare blood cancer, myelofibrosis, when she was seventy-two. After being hospitalized three times in one year with pneumonia, she could not sustain the barrage of attacks on her body.

Rob had been particularly close to my mom, one of those truly joyful people who know the difference between problems and inconveniences. They were Scrabble buddies, compulsively neat, and while neither of them was good at cooking, I appreciated that both she and Rob would clean up after I made a meal. Mom had a condo in Atlanta and an apartment in Manhattan, where she was a freelance tour guide. We had a close friendship like no other, and she relished being "Bebe," grandmother to our children, River and Skye, as well as Zoe and Griffin, those of my brother, Scott. and his wife, Amy.

Immediately after Mom's death, Rob's liver disease, which was "at bay" through medication, began to worsen. When I look back on the months when Mom was in and out of the hospital, I realize I could not have taken care of both of them at the same time.

That summer, Rob's appearance began to change dramatically. His skin and eyes became yellow (jaundiced), his face began to hollow, and his body thinned from muscle-mass wasting. He was itchy from the inside out, fatigued, and clearly in more immediate need of a liver transplant. By August, with his health rapidly deteriorating, I banned him from going out on our charters aboard the *Royal Princess* after he jumped off the boat onto the dock with his legs collapsing. Luckily, we had an excellent crew at that time, especially Rob's brother, Marco, who could handle virtually anything mechanical, and his Italian-born wife, Maria, my beloved sister-in-law, who was our awesome head chef.

For the first time, Rob and I switched roles, and I saw our business from a different perspective. Suddenly, I fully realized how much responsibility Rob took on between Coast Guard inspections, mechanical maintenance, and overseeing every detail during the charters. I had handled sales and event planning by phone, allowing me to work from home and be close by for the children. Rob traveled over an hour each way for showings and charters. After booking and coordinating events, I would pass the event summaries to the yacht staff for execution, rarely going out on the charters. Rob preferred to be the captain in charge on the vessel, but lately, I would hear comments from various employees that he looked particularly worn out or frequently lost his temper. He took pride in every detail, but the physical and emotional stress was becoming too much for him.

So he began staying home with the kids while I was onboard every charter overseeing the events, greeting guests, working with the staff and crew. Although it was a lot of physical work, I enjoyed being there watching people celebrate momentous moments in their lives.

Meanwhile, Rob and I had been exploring his options for having a liver transplant. We eventually learned that the chances of getting a deceased donor liver more quickly would be far greater in Florida than in New York. You would think that since the Northeast has a more concentrated population, there would be more donors, but it was not the case. We were not exactly sure why. Were people less likely to sign up to be donors in the Northeast? Or was the transplant system better coordinated in other regions?

Rob had been a liver disease patient at Montefiore Hospital in the Bronx for a while. He had a good relationship with his hepatologist, Dr. Sam Sigal, but once he was put on the transplant list, Rob felt that one of the transplant surgeons he met with was too aggressive.

In New York, the median Model End Stage Liver Disease (MELD) score, which determines priority on the liver transplant waitlist, was very high, averaging thirty-five—at which point a patient is considered very close to mortality; a score of forty is the highest. The MELD score is based on blood levels, measuring liver and kidney functions.

Although Rob's liver counts were high enough to be listed, he was only at a score of seventeen, so his chances of getting a transplant in New York were low. He could not get a higher priority on the regional transplant list unless he became extremely sick and was hospitalized twice in three months; this could give him exception points to raise his MELD score.

A living donor is a person who passes a strict medical and psychological evaluation and agrees to donate fifty percent of their liver to someone in need; afterward, the donor's and the recipient's livers would regenerate to their normal size. At Montefiore, we were encouraged to find a living donor. PSC patients like Rob often suffer longer with fatigue, jaundice, and other complications even though their MELD score does not always reflect how sick they are. We felt trapped, and a living donor could be a quicker solution. But nothing is without risk, and, contrary to the name of his first live-aboard boat, *Risk it All*, Rob was never keen on having anyone risk their own life for him with this surgery.

The Montefiore request for a living donor prompted me to set up a Facebook page in 2018 dedicated to finding a liver match for Rob. For me, finally "letting the secret out of the bag" was cathartic. I needed to feel less isolated, and I began using social media to help both of us. My husband has always been private about his disease, but not being able to freely talk about it had been restrictive for me. His doctor said, "Rob, you don't get any points by being too private. You need a new liver. Tell everyone you know."

We found two potential donors, one of whom was a great match—Josh, brother-in-law of Rob's niece Stephanie. Josh had the same blood type as Rob, was a similar size, and wanted to do this for him. Both men served in the armed forces and perhaps felt a shared camaraderie. Josh went through the strict evaluation process but was rejected. While the hospital did not tell us the reason, we felt sure it was because he had post-traumatic stress disorder (PTSD) from serving in Iraq, and that perhaps the transplant team feared the surgery might trigger a PTSD episode. Josh wrote an excellent letter to the committee explaining that he was now married and in a mentally stable place. Furious about the situation, I began looking at another transplant hospital in New York that might reconsider having him as the donor.

The other potential living donor was a distant cousin of Rob's through his father's family. Teresa, who won the Miss America contest in 2011 and had also served in the U.S. Air Force, was the mother of a young child. Rob did not want anyone with children going through the evaluation, especially a single mother.

At our Montefiore evaluation, I remember asking if there was a liver transplant support group and being frustrated to find they did not have anything that met on a regular basis. It felt like we were our own leaf on a branch of a tree, not knowing where the trunk or the roots were grounded.

Rob has always trusted his gut. He is a numbers guy. While Montefiore had a good reputation of outcome after surgery, the staff had a small number of liver transplant surgeons performing an average of forty liver transplants a year.

After doing extensive research with websites like www.srtr.org (Scientific Registry of Transplant Recipients), Rob learned that the

Mayo Clinic in Jacksonville, Florida, did an average of 170 liver transplants per year and had six full-time abdominal transplant surgeons. He became laser-focused with a file about two inches thick containing printouts from different hospitals around the country with their statistics, including average MELD scores for transplants, number performed per year, and survival rates.

"Would you take your specialty car to be fixed at a regular automotive shop?" Rob would ask me. "Or would you take it to where they do this on a more regular basis?"

And so, in September 2019, Rob set up evaluation appointments at Mayo Clinic in the midst of our crazy fall yacht-chartering schedule. Together we went to Jacksonville for a week leaving our business in the hands of our capable crew and our kids in the hands of Marco and Maria.

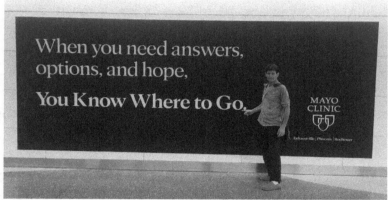

September 2019, Rob at Jacksonville airport before visiting Mayo Clinic

CHAPTER 5

Our Big Move

September 2019, Jacksonville, Florida

Heading south, we first flew from Newark to Atlanta to see my brother, Scott, and my witty, intelligent, idealist father, who was now in a wheelchair with severe dementia and round-the-clock in-home care.

We drove from Atlanta to Jacksonville, where we spent a week at Mayo Clinic being interviewed by and meeting with members of the transplant team. We also had to attend educational classes from departments within the Mayo Clinic, including a hepatologist, surgeon, nutritionist, social worker, psychologist, and liver coordinator. The team needed to assess if Rob was a good transplant candidate and had the support he needed afterwards. Years ago, even though it was more expensive, I made sure we had health insurance that did not limit us to receiving care only in the state we lived in.

Both of us were blown away by the entire organization at Mayo. Not only was the facility immaculate, set on lovely grounds with fountains, flowers, walkways, and an onsite hotel, but the staff members were friendly, took their time, and provided almost immediate testing results.

With Rob's bile duct disease, we also learned from one of the surgeons we met with that living donor transplant (LDT) surgeries are more complicated because you are connecting smaller vessels.

With a disorder like PSC, it made sense to me that it would be smoother to connect the main bile duct of a deceased donor liver to the recipient's remaining bile duct or re-route the donor's large bile duct to the recipient's intestine instead of re-creating a bile duct from a living donor's remaining liver.

I had been devastated when our potential living donor at Montefiore was not approved, but in retrospect, I believe the LDT surgery would not have been optimal for Rob. We were accepted into the Mayo program with the condition that Rob live preferably within an hour from the hospital while waiting for a transplant.

Not only did Rob feel confident in the Mayo Clinic, he also realized that in New York, he could be risking complications or death before an organ was available. We already knew the importance of MELD scores; the higher the number, the sicker a person is. The average score for transplant in Florida was twenty-six, compared to New York's figure of thirty-five.

Being proactive, it didn't take long for Rob to decide that he should temporarily relocate to Florida while the kids and I would remain in Nyack through the school year, visiting him during breaks. If he got the transplant call, I would immediately fly down to be with him. Our fifteen-year-old son, River, was in the ninth grade and thriving on the travel soccer team. Skye was in her last year of elementary school. We wanted to keep their lives as normal as possible.

While going through the week-long Mayo Clinic evaluation, we took a day trip to historic St. Augustine, only forty-five minutes south of Jacksonville, and loved it. There are daily trolley tours, museums, narrow streets, great restaurants, and the scenic Flagler College. We knew instantly that was where Rob should live. After searching online, he found a three-bedroom condo with a pier and boat slip on Anastasia Island, across the Bridge of Lions from downtown St. Augustine. As he would need a temporary caregiver, he asked a childhood friend, who was suddenly single and retiring, if he wanted to join him.

In a few weeks, Rob had our twenty-seven-foot Ranger tugboat, *Andiamo*, sent by trailer down along with his scooter. If he was going to live there awhile, he would try to make it fun, especially when we were there together. Things were falling into place. So, in late October, after a goodbye party, Rob and his friend drove down and arrived in St. Augustine to begin a new chapter.

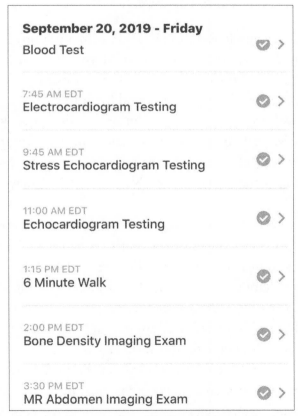

September 20, 2019 - Friday
Blood Test

7:45 AM EDT
Electrocardiogram Testing

9:45 AM EDT
Stress Echocardiogram Testing

11:00 AM EDT
Echocardiogram Testing

1:15 PM EDT
6 Minute Walk

2:00 PM EDT
Bone Density Imaging Exam

3:30 PM EDT
MR Abdomen Imaging Exam

Snapshot from one day of Rob's transplant evaluation

CHAPTER 6

The First 'Dry Run'

November 2019, Jacksonville

"Hi, I'm Captain Rob, and I'm here with my family. I have been on the liver transplant list at Mayo Clinic since October. We live in Nyack, New York, but I am here because the list is shorter in Florida, and also this hospital is world renowned."

This was how Rob introduced himself at the Tuesday morning meeting of Mayo Clinic's Second Chance Support Group for liver and kidney transplant patients and their caregivers. During the Thanksgiving school break, River, Skye, and I had flown down to Florida.

Rob, who had been counting the days until we arrived, had waited for us to visit all the local tourist attractions. We wanted it to feel like a mini family vacation, but we also took the kids to the Mayo support group meeting for a better understanding of our true purpose in being there. To ease their fears and answer their questions, we wanted the kids to see the hospital and know there are many people who are thriving after transplants.

Social worker Mike Womack led the support group sessions, where people sat in a circle talking in a private room. There were usually about twelve regulars in the group. Afterwards, those interested would go out to lunch together, which was organized by Kristin, wife of transplant patient Steve.

"Hello, everyone," Mike began each meeting. "I'd like you all to introduce yourselves and let us know if you are either pre- or post-transplant or a caregiver. This is a time to ask questions or share something relevant to the rest of the group."

Pre-transplant patients usually asked questions, while post-transplant patients were eager to answer and tell their stories. While most of the group were locals at that time, often transplant recipients would attend the group when they were back for Mayo visits.

Many months later, Rob would describe his experience in an interview. "I was put on the active waitlist October 21, 2019. They told me to have my cell phone with me at all times and answer every call even if I did not recognize the number," he said. "When I first came down here, I tried to do as much as I could to stay active but was getting more and more fatigued. Basically, I was just waiting for a call while going once a week to the support group at Mayo Clinic, which gave me something to look forward to."

Rob had been to a few meetings before we got there, and he felt comfortable. He was one of a few pre-transplant patients in the group. He told me how welcoming everyone was and especially bonded with Andy and his wife, Gloria, Toosie, Lynn, Jerry, and John and his wife, Trink. This made me happy because he was developing a community.

Not having seen him for a month, I immediately noticed the difference in Rob's appearance. He was even more jaundiced, meaning the whites of his eyes and skin tone were yellow, and he had lost a considerable amount of muscle mass. While our lives were going on as usual in New York, the toughest part for Rob was being separated from us, wasting away while missing his family.

A man with exceedingly good taste, Rob had picked the perfect place for us. Our second-level unit had a spacious back deck overlooking the courtyard, palm trees, pool, flat, calm bay, and private pier leading out to docks where *Andiamo* was tied up. We ate many of our meals together watching porpoises and the quiet state park beach in the distance.

The route from the condo to Jacksonville was beautiful. I loved the Spanish moss hanging down from the oak trees. Each time we went to Mayo, our drive took us through St. Augustine's historic old town, passing the Castillo de San Marcos on our right overlooking Matanzas Bay, and then over the Vilano Bridge, which rises and descends overlooking the Intracoastal Waterway on each side with the sunrise and ocean in the distance. Heading north on A1A through Vilano Beach, with Guana River State Park on our left, into Ponte Vedra. We took Butler Boulevard and crossed another bridge with views of the St. Johns River, to the San Pablo exit where we would see the Mayo Clinic building in the distance.

After our first visit to St. Augustine as a family, it was hard to leave. On December 3, I was flying back to Newark Airport with the kids, with a short layover. When the plane landed for the Atlanta connection, I saw a text from Rob. He'd gotten a call from Mayo's Procurement office and was on his way to the hospital.

They had a possible liver for him but would not know for sure until the surgeons inspected it. While it was considered a high-risk, hepatitis C liver, doctors had assured us that today, hepatitis C can be almost totally cured through medication after transplant.

We did not expect a call so soon. I wasn't sure what to do. Should I turn around and fly back to Jacksonville alone, sending the kids on to New York without me? The airlines said I had to fill out a bunch of paperwork, which we did not have time for, so I continued on, anxious to know what was happening.

We landed in Newark, and our friend Jonathan picked us up and drove us to Nyack. He planned to spend the night on our sofa, ready to take me back to the airport if the surgery was happening.

At midnight, Rob called and said that the surgeons halted the operation once they inspected the liver first-hand. Apparently, it wasn't working properly. This experience we now know is called a "dry run," and it is somewhat common.

I used to think that if someone died from an accident on the side of the road, someone could scoop them up and use their organs for transplant. Nope. The person's body has to still be "alive," but their brain has to be "dead." The potential donor has to be hooked up to machines in a hospital, with the okay from the family to procure their organs after it has been confirmed that there is absolutely no chance the donor will survive. Then, hospitals make procurement calls from the long waiting list of people.

Rob returned to the condo that night with mixed emotions. For the next several months, the support group meetings were invaluable to his morale. He was waiting and ready for his second chance. I found out later that when receiving the first call, Rob thought about another member of the support group who appeared much sicker than him, and he asked if the liver could go to her instead; however, he was the best match for this one. The on-call procurement coordinator told Rob that in all the years working, she had never had a patient make this request to forfeit an organ on behalf of another patient.

At Mayo, those who have been through the transplant tunnel share their experiences, giving confidence and hope to people in the beginning process, as we were. After interviewing transplant patients for this book, a few commonalities have struck me. First, there is an eagerness and joy in telling their stories. There is sheer gratitude for being alive with a newfound appreciation of each moment and a desire to help others. I have been amazed by these seemingly unremarkable people with remarkable stories. Many of these individuals have become our living angels.

One is Andy, who had his own transplant in 2007. When Rob arrived, Andy took him under his wing and checked in on him frequently, with watchfulness and encouragement.

Another unforgettable friend is Toosie, who lives in Ponte Vedra Beach. When Rob first came down to St. Augustine, he attended a potluck dinner for support group members at Toosie's home, and she and her husband, Denny, were so welcoming to him. Rob felt he was part of a special family of transplant recipients who embraced him.

Andy's and Toosie's stories are shared in the following chapters.

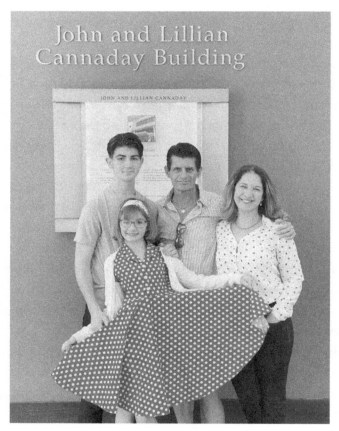

The Bellanich family just after attending
Mayo Clinic Second Chance Support group

CHAPTER 7

Andy and Gloria: 'Back to Sanity'

One of the insidious by-products of end-stage liver disease is encephalopathy. This can develop when the liver stops filtering ammonia out of the body, which affects the brain's ability to function properly. Patients with encephalopathy may experience severe cognitive side effects, such as an altered level of consciousness or confusion that can be disturbing and dangerous. In Andy's case, his wife, Gloria, was there with him every step of the way. Together, they made it through that dark time and want others to know there are important signals for a caregiver or loved one to look for.

"I don't remember a lot of what happened right before my transplant," Andy told me. "You'd have to ask Gloria. I often say that the harder job is not the patient's but the caregiver's." He knows that in some circumstances, a patient may not realize how bad things are. "I remember ... waking up in places and not knowing how I had gotten there. That's when I started wearing a medical alert tag so people wouldn't think I was drunk or mentally ill."

"Yes, Andy will often ask me to recount things that have happened, and I've always been honest with him because it also helps him understand my side of things," Gloria interjected. "On one trip to the hospital, Andy tried to jump out of the car. When we arrived, he told the nurse he did not know who these people were, meaning me and our son. Meanwhile, I was still trying to process all of this."

During Andy's illness, Gloria was also going back and forth between their home in St. Augustine and Tallahassee, where her father was ill; he died shortly before Andy's transplant in 2007. "I felt nervous leaving Andy alone because he would get so confused and even get physical. He would sleep most of the day and be up most of the night," she said. "We had a password. If I called him and he did not know the password, I knew he was in trouble. When he didn't answer the phone at all, that concerned me even more, and I'd ask a neighbor to go check on him. We had to take his car keys away because one day he drove north like a crazy man towards the Florida-Georgia line, then had no idea how he had gotten there."

Andy, born in 1953, grew up in the farmlands of Hammonton, New Jersey, and joined the U.S. Navy. He was stationed at Mayport in Jacksonville, Florida. A hull tech, firefighter, and welder, he served aboard the USS Sarsfield, and in late '73, the ship docked in Genoa, Italy. Maybe it was something he had eaten or drunk, but Andy developed hepatitis A and became extremely sick with sweats, chills, jaundice, and hallucinations. He spent three weeks in a ward in a local hospital, a fifteenth-century building, where he had transfusions and IVs. Eventually he was transferred to a military hospital in Germany, then sent home. Years later, the Mayo Clinic traced the Genoa hospital as the place Andy contracted hepatitis C.

After the Navy years, he married and had two sons. When the marriage ended, Andy became a full-custody single dad with a five-and a six-year-old. He was working at his own construction company, and when the boys were twelve and thirteen, he met Gloria, who was nurturing and easy to be with. His sons sat Andy down and said, "Dad, here's the deal. You either marry Gloria, or we're kicking you out of the house!" They married in 1992.

Life was good, full of outdoor activities, fulfilling work, weddings, then grandchildren. Many times, someone with a liver disease has no idea there is a problem until something else occurs making it apparent that the liver cannot do its job.

"I was at a family get-together in 2001," Andy recalled. "Maybe it was the ice cream or the barbecue, but suddenly I got sick. My stomach issues turned out to be my gallbladder. When all the blood work came back, we were informed that I had hepatitis C. During my gallbladder surgery, they did a liver biopsy, which came back positive for cirrhosis. After five years of treatments and hospitalizations, we were sent to the Mayo Clinic. In 2006, Mayo informed us that I had cancer of the liver."

"Andy was covered under my health insurance policy from my job at Coastal Construction Products," Gloria explained. "But there was a clause that excluded coverage for liver transplants. Because he was a veteran, we were trying to get him approved for VA benefits, but the process was taking too long. He needed a transplant immediately. The big boss pulled me into his office one day and told me to sit down. For a moment, I thought I was being fired. He asked me to tell him everything that was going on with Andy and to give him the names of his doctors. A week later, my other boss told me they had contacted Mayo and personally guaranteed payment for all of Andy's care, including a liver transplant. 'We are a family-oriented business,' he said. 'We have got to take care of our employees.'"

Three weeks later, Andy's MELD score shot up into the mid-forties, a score so high that most people do not survive. Gloria could barely recount the story without tearing up. "At our next appointment, the doctor wanted to admit Andy, but there were no beds available, so we had to go home. Andy's encephalopathy was the worst it had ever been. At 2:30 a.m. he woke me up, standing at our bedroom door repeating, 'I stubbed my toe. I stubbed my toe.' I said, 'Andy, you're six feet away from the bed.'

"Andy kept repeating himself, and when he shook me hard by the shoulders, I knew he was not in his right mind. I called 911 and told them that Andy was waiting on a liver transplant and had encephalopathy."

When the paramedics, police, and firemen got to the house, they assured Gloria they had dealt with this before. As they approached Andy lying in his bed, he started swinging at them. He took on five paramedics and two police officers, but they finally got him on a gurney and in the ambulance. The next day when he woke up in the hospital, Andy became aggressive again; after being tied to the bed, he tried to chew one of his restraints off. Doctors decided his situation was so serious that they intubated and put him into a coma. Andy had been in the coma three days when Mayo Clinic notified Gloria that they had a liver for him. His condition would not interfere with the surgery, doctors felt. But after an all-night wait at the hospital, the transplant had to be called off because when the surgeons fully inspected the liver, it was not satisfactory.

After being in a coma in the ICU for sixteen days, Andy was transferred into a regular room for another five days. When Gloria was told he was being discharged, she argued with the doctor, saying Andy was not in his right mind and should not be at home. But at that point, there was no medical reason to keep him there.

Gloria had a tough time taking care of him, and one weekend her sons told her to go spend the night with a friend, and they would take over, giving her a break. That Saturday, March 24, 2007, after dropping Andy off at a store to meet his sons, she took her car to get the oil changed. Not fifteen minutes later, Andy called her saying, "I have to go to the hospital. I have to go to the hospital." After repeating this several minutes, he told her, "I got a call from Mayo. They may have a liver for me."

She hurried to meet Andy at the hospital. "Even after thirteen years, I get emotional when I think back to that night when they finally told me that the surgery was a go," Gloria recounted as her eyes filled with tears. "They let me go back as they were wheeling him into the operating room. Andy looked back at me as if to say, 'It's finally over.' He was so sick. I was so scared. The doctors assured me everything was going to be okay."

The surgery lasted about five hours, and Andy was transferred to the ICU. "The next morning when I saw him, I was shocked," Gloria said. "They already had him sitting up in a chair, and the whites of his eyes were white again, not yellow. His skin was already back to a normal color. I turned around and looked at the doctor like, 'Are you friggin' kidding me?' The doctor smiled and gave me the thumbs-up. I couldn't believe in that short number of hours he had changed so quickly."

Three months after the surgery, a complication arose with an artery that had been placed over Andy's urethra during the transplant. Surgeons went back in laparoscopically to rearrange the urethra, inserting a stent that remained for six weeks. "I experienced what it must be like to go to the gynecologist," Andy said with a laugh. "They had to put me in a room with stirrups to remove the stent. How do women go through this every year? I have never been so embarrassed in all my life."

Andy's compromised immune system may have been an issue when he developed tonsil cancer ten years after his transplant, shocking both him and Gloria. "You get to a point where you have been through so much, then things are going so well that it was completely unexpected," she recalled. "Andy had to go through chemo, then radiation. He asked me not to treat him like an invalid throughout the process because he had felt like one during the transplant."

At Gloria's retirement party from Coastal in 2018, she stood in front of her colleagues and said to her bosses, "I can never repay you or thank you enough for saving my husband's life. I know Andy would not be here today if it weren't for you."

Rob and I felt blessed to have this couple in our lives, especially during the long months when Rob waited in St. Augustine, far from his family. A steadfast friend, Andy called regularly to check on him and offer companionship. He invited Rob to cowboy quick-draw shooting competitions and even accompanied him to Miami for a boat show on Valentine's Day in 2020.

Andy and Gloria hadn't had a support group before his transplant, and they wish they had. "Seeing how many others are going through or have gone through this makes me feel part of a family. I have spoken a lot about encephalopathy in our group, and it has helped other caregivers recognize the signs. Sharing my story helps give information and hope to others who are waiting. Life can get back to a new normal," Gloria said confidently.

"My life has been great," Andy declared. "We have seen three more grandkids and one great-grandson born since my transplant. I'm thankful every morning I wake up. I believe you gotta give back multiple times what you've gotten. If I hear someone getting down and talking about wanting to go meet their maker, I shake them up a bit. There is life after transplant, and it is wonderful."

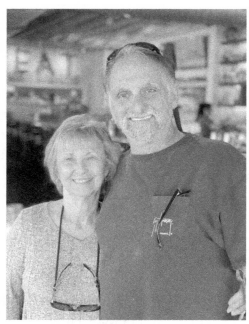

Andy and Gloria, February 2020 after support
group luncheon

CHAPTER 8

Toosie: Finding Her Donor

Another support group member and friend is Toosie, proud mother of three daughters and grandmother of fourteen grandchildren, who has become a spokesperson for organ donation programs since her liver transplant in 2017.

"Not everyone wants to meet their donor family," Toosie acknowledged. "And not every donor family wants to meet the person who is living with the organ of their loved one. In my case, I was fortunate to meet mine."

An organ recipient is allowed to write a generic letter to their donor family four months after a transplant. It has to be approved by their transplant center with certain criteria. Just as with an adoption, there is a shroud of secrecy between the two camps unless both parties want to know about each other. So, after her transplant, Toosie wrote a letter to her unknown donor family thanking them, which was then sent to the organ procurement organization via the Mayo Clinic. She enclosed a picture of herself, her husband, Denny, and their grandchildren at the beach—all wearing matching green shirts that displayed the words "Team Toosie."

A few months later, her oldest daughter, Melissa, posted that same photo on her Twitter account. Miraculously, the sister of Toosie's donor recognized the picture and contacted Melissa. The connection prompted the families to meet for coffee, leading to tears and honest conversation. Toosie learned the name and details of her donor, who had died of suicide at age thirty-six, having battled a twelve-year opioid addiction after a fall that injured his back.

"When you meet your donor family, you face yourself," Toosie confessed. "Whatever judgments you may have about people, it is right in front of you. Ultimately, my life went on because of this man's gift."

Before her transplant, she and Denny were living in Tallahassee, their days full of family, friends, volunteering, church, running marathons, enjoying sports, the beach and long walks. They attended almost every event that went on in their grandchildren's lives.

She was being treated for fatty liver disease, and for years, the doctors at the hospital watched her numbers, which became elevated in 2017. "I was told that women process alcohol differently from men, and I certainly processed alcohol very differently! I cut back, but did not quit. Mine was a combination of alcohol, fatty liver, and overuse of antibiotics through the years."

Her ordeal began after a leg wound when she pulled an azalea bush too hard; the liver condition prevented the wound from healing, and sepsis developed. She spent the month of October 2017 in a hospital, and doctors told her family to call in hospice. They did not offer transplant as an option.

"If it weren't for my private gastroenterologist, Dr. Rodriguez, I would not be here today," she said. "He told us that a transplant could be a real option in the future. He gave us hope. 'If it were me,' he told us, 'I would go to the Mayo Clinic where your family support is.'"

Her husband and daughters decided to "hijack" Toosie from the hospital in Tallahassee. They made insurance changes, contacted Mayo, and transported her to their Ponte Vedra Beach condo. "On Halloween night, I watched my grandchildren come into the house, but I was barely conscious," Toosie said. "I ended up going by emergency ambulance to Mayo, was admitted that evening, and placed in the ICU with a critical condition."

Toosie's insurance was to switch at 12:01 a.m., November 1, her sixty-seventh birthday. Her evaluation process for transplant began November 3, but she has no memory of it due to severe encephalopathy.

"On November 13, I received my gift," Toosie said quietly. "Three weeks later, I was sent to Brooks Rehab to learn to walk, write, and dress and feed myself again. My caregivers were Denny, our daughters, and my sisters, who came from different areas to sit with me. Fortunately, I was not left alone for one minute. Denny has been my rock and theirs! Since I was a stay-at-home mom and Denny was working in law enforcement, my girls considered me as the family nurturer. They saw a side of their father they hadn't seen before, and it brought us even closer."

At first, Toosie did not want to attend the Mayo support group because she never felt she needed to have others aid her in dealing with situations; she was strong and had lots of will power. "But now, I enjoy the group," she said. "It is informative, and I feel that if there is one scared person who comes through those doors, I might help them see it is not so scary, nor the end of one's life."

Today, her days go much as they did before—family, friends, church, exercise, and moving on. "It is just a different adventure with pills involved. Also, I spend time volunteering. A woman in organ procurement schedules me to speak at high schools to teenagers getting their driver's license so that they are educated about organ transplant. I simply tell my story. It's up to them whether or not they want to check the box indicating they choose to be a donor. We try and dispel some of the myths. Many people are afraid to check that box thinking that doctors will not do everything possible to save their life. That is not true," she emphasized.

"Mayo is my safe place. It is a balancing act between donor and recipient. Now, I have trust in Mayo and the Lord. They are looking after me. They want success for me and for my donor's family to know something very good came from their gift after their tragic loss."

A week or so after I wrote Toosie's story, she texted me something that she forgot to mention. "Right before my transplant, I was hallucinating, but I remember seeing three angels," she told me. "Perhaps they represented my three daughters."

"No," I said definitively. "My medium friend, Susan, says that when you die, three of your angels who have passed are there watching over you." When my own mother was in the hospital various times before her death in 2019, Susan had told me how many angels she saw on each occasion. She knew my mother had died on May 4 because she saw three angels, and I shared this with Toosie.

"Technically, you died," I said, "but then you were brought back to life with a new liver." Toosie had chills.

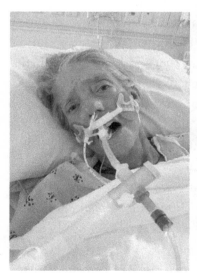
Toosie in the hospital

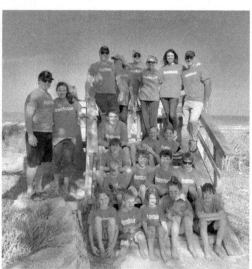
Toosie and her family

CHAPTER 9

Quarantined During a Pandemic

March 2020, St. Augustine

Wearing masks and gloves, I boarded a United flight in Newark on March 20 with my children and only a handful of other passengers. When we landed at the Jacksonville airport, Rob picked us up, and we went straight to the condo in St. Augustine to quarantine.

The coronavirus, COVID-19, had hit New York in mid-March like a tidal wave. A few cases turned into hundreds, then thousands, and it became a nightmare. Schools were suddenly closed, and students had to continue their learning online, while social distancing was encouraged to avoid getting sick.

Rob wanted us to come to Florida right away, which made logical sense. However, I was nervous that we might be exposing him to the virus. Many of my friends warned us to "get out while you can." So I bought three one-way tickets to Jacksonville with no idea how long we would stay, whether our NYC yacht chartering business would stay afloat, or whether we might harm Rob's chances of getting a transplant.

Within days after we left, restrictions on traveling were implemented, and cases of the virus had overloaded New York's healthcare system. We were experiencing the unimaginable—a worldwide pandemic. Businesses like ours were abruptly shut down. Restaurants could open only for take-out. Our economy and normal way of life were at a standstill. In retrospect, if Mom had lived another year, she might not have even gotten a bed in the ICU due to this pandemic.

Conversely, the paradox was that while we were scared and physically isolated from each other, it also forced us to be present in the moment. We had to let go of what we could not control and accept what was happening. Life slowed down. This, I thought, might be affecting whether or not Rob could get a healthy liver transplant in time. Our children were unhappy about leaving home, but we needed to be together as a family.

Since last fall, Rob had been eagerly attending the Second Chance Support Group meetings. After the COVID-19 outbreak, no one was able to freely go to the Mayo Clinic, so our social worker, Mike, began scheduling virtual meetings on the Zoom platform, the new way of bringing people together. While this helped, along with a private Second Chance Facebook group, video didn't replace the face-to-face contact, but the benefit was that people in other locations now could participate.

The support group was and still is a tight-knit community, and members feel like family. Some people come to Mayo for a short period of time and may attend the group only a few times because they live elsewhere. Others, who were already local or relocated here while waiting, attend regularly.

Once we escaped New York for Florida, I sat next to Rob every Tuesday morning participating in the virtual meetings. It was important. We needed it.

Outside the meetings, we formed a special bond with transplant patient Jerry. His survival story was extraordinary, and his positive outlook on life was fabulous.

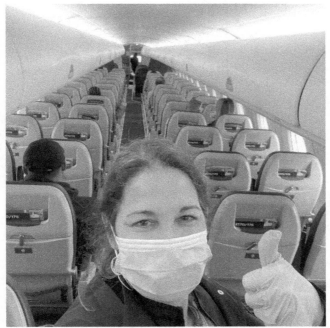

Lezlee and kids escape New York during the beginning of the pandemic

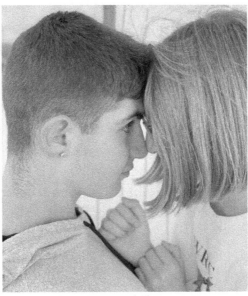

River and Skye

CHAPTER 10

Jerry and His 'Sassy Liver'

"Jerry, why do you think you have a sassy liver?" I asked this witty, upbeat man almost three years after his liver transplant.

"Well, I think I have a sassy liver because after surgery, I started craving pedicures, and I never wanted anyone to touch my feet before," he replied with his slightly Southern accent. "Then, according to my brother, A.J., I was very snappy and demanding, so we nicknamed it my sassy liver. It's so crazy because now I crave foods that I never ate before, like crab legs with Tabasco sauce and melted butter."

Before the transplant, Jerry was always on the go, out seven nights a week socializing, attending performances or board meetings of performing arts organizations. He owned properties in Florida, Las Vegas, and New York City, produced Broadway musicals, and owned a 17,000-square-foot gay bar/nightclub with his brother in Jacksonville.

"Just before Jerry's transplant," A.J. said, "we went to London for ten days. I could not keep up with my brother, who kept going from early morning until late in the evening. I always called him 'Jerry on the run.'"

Jerry, the youngest of three children, grew up in a conservative Jewish family in Jacksonville. His father, who traveled a lot on business, looked forward to coming home and spending time with his family, and his mother owned a health food store.

At eighteen years old, Jerry had never been out of the state of Florida and yearned to travel. He bought his first rental property, renovated it, and kept going. From then on, he traveled internationally and cherished his many friendships.

He had no idea that he had any health problems. Along with overseeing the Jacksonville nightclub, he spent one week a month in his New York City apartment and went to Las Vegas frequently for trade shows. After his brother's divorce, they bought a home together in Jacksonville with plenty of space to have their own privacy. Jerry was on top of the world—until it almost came crashing down.

On April 6, 2017, he and a cousin left on a Princess cruise headed for Bermuda, Ireland, England, and France. The ship was five hours late leaving port in Fort Lauderdale due to a bomb threat, so it was after 9 p.m. when they sailed. Deciding it was too late to go to the dining room for dinner, Jerry suggested they go with the buffet that evening. "I didn't realize the food had been sitting out for five hours waiting for us to be cleared to leave, and I ate something that made me very sick," he told me.

The next morning, even more ill, he went to the ship's infirmary. "They had me call A.J. in Florida and tell him that I had food poisoning. They were making me get off the ship on Sunday in Bermuda. My brother said to keep in touch with him, and he would come and meet me and help me get home.

"The next thing I knew, I woke up on a stretcher in an air ambulance landing in Fort Lauderdale. Suddenly, I realized that it was the following Tuesday, and I had been in a coma all that time."

When the Bermuda hospital had contacted his brother, A.J. tried desperately to get a plane ticket to go there, but due to holidays and a bad storm, he could not get a flight out. And the main goal was to get Jerry back to the United States. "Finally, I posted a request for help on Facebook, and a friend, Becky, reached out. She helped arrange the air ambulance service after I was pleading for someone to get Jerry on that plane," A.J. recalled. Without hesitation, he put down his credit card for the $38,000 fee.

Doctors had told him that Jerry had a zero percent chance of survival in the Bermuda hospital, and if an air ambulance flew him home, his chance of survival was still less than one percent. "They thought I could die when the plane changed altitude during landing," Jerry said. "My brother took the risk and hired the air ambulance. When the plane's altitude decreased, and we were landing, I woke up. What a blessing!

"No one really knew what was wrong with me, and the only place that would accept me was the Cleveland Clinic in Weston, Florida."

Another friend of theirs, Patrick, had helped by calling hospitals all over Florida. "I was getting terribly agitated feeling like I was talking to a wall when I talked to hospital operators," said A.J., who drove six hours to meet Jerry at the Cleveland Clinic.

During the next twenty-four hours, Jerry found out that he had a fatty liver that would not process the food poisoning. "At first, I thought my liver would rejuvenate itself; I would do everything I could to be healthy to make that happen," he said. "But my mind frame began changing after I received a phone call from a close friend, singer Tony Orlando, who told me that six of his friends had had successful liver transplants. He made me promise him that I would do everything I could to get a transplant to save my life."

A.J. remembered how stressful and worrying that time was. "Honestly, I didn't understand a lot of what the doctors were saying. They were talking about his bilirubin levels, but I thought they were talking about a Reuben sandwich! When I heard the words 'liver transplant,' I knew it would be better if we were closer to home. The only way the doctors would release Jerry was if we went straight to the emergency room at Mayo Clinic."

The following week when Jerry was able to travel, they made arrangements to do just that. "It was the best decision of my life,"

Jerry said emphatically. From the ER in Jacksonville, he was sent home, and the next morning, Mayo called to start his testing and evaluation for transplant.

The next week, Jerry got very sick and was admitted to the hospital. Afterwards, he was in and out of a coma. "The head of Mayo Clinic visited me at the end of April, assuring me that they would do all they could to help me get a new liver and survive."

On May 7, 2017, he received his new, "sassy" liver. "I didn't realize I had had a liver transplant until my brother told me the next day. That's how sick I was," he said. "I was in the hospital nearly three weeks after surgery, in a rehab facility for three weeks, and another week in a nursing home before I could come home."

"I was scared every day for three months, especially when Jerry was in and out of comas," A.J. confessed. "Once the transplant was over and he went to rehab, I told him that I wasn't going to wheel him around or take him to the bathroom because I knew he could walk. 'No pain, no gain.' We are fighters."

Today, other than lots of medications every day and frequent blood work and testing, things are back to normal for Jerry. "I am involved in two wonderful support groups at Mayo, and I love volunteering with transplant patients and their caregivers, and speaking to a lot of organizations about the importance of organ transplantation. You can't take your organs with you. Helping someone else is the last unselfish thing you can do in your life."

In 2018, he participated in the Transplant Games of America in Salt Lake City, and the next year in the World Transplant Games in Newcastle, England. "These were huge challenges for me. I've met some of the greatest people in the world, people who have been through many of the same challenges that I have. Surprisingly, I won a Gold Medal at the World Games for bowling!" Jerry also felt honored to be part of setting a Guinness world record in Salt Lake City for being among the largest number of transplant recipients in one gathering space.

"I thank God every day for this opportunity of a second chance at life. My mission now is to simply give back. That's why I am so involved with support groups and everything else I am doing."

An amazing turn came in October 2020, when a longtime bar manager at Jerry's nightclub had an unexpected injury causing him to become brain-dead. Clarence had been proud of his decision to be an organ donor, and his organs ended up going to people in need. Jerry, along with Clarence's mother and sisters, participated in the heartbreaking yet reverent "honor walk" that doctors made to transfer the body into the operating room before procurement. Hospital staff lined the aisles in silence. Later, Jerry coordinated the funeral service at the club for his employee and friend.

"Having inside me someone else's liver that has saved my life, and then experiencing my friend's death, which led to his ultimate gift as an organ donor, all of this has made me even more committed to advocating on behalf of organ donation and transplantation," Jerry said. "My story has come full circle."

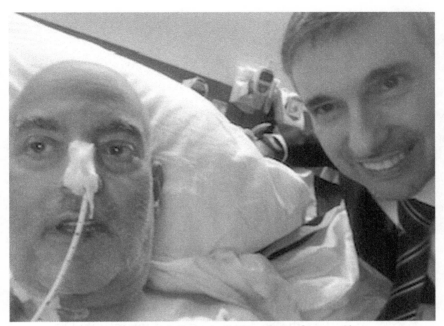

Jerry with Gianrico Farrugia, M.D., CEO of Mayo Clinic

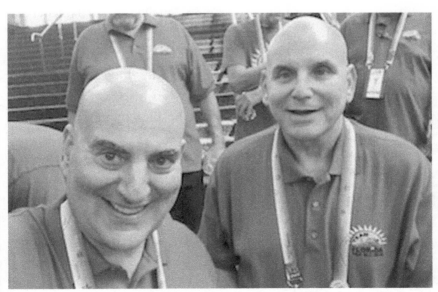

Jerry and AJ at the Transplant Games of America in Salt Lake City, Utah

CHAPTER 11

Our Experience Being the Backup Recipient

April 2020, St. Augustine

We were all set to go out on the boat Saturday morning, April 4, to explore the St. Johns River. A thought came over me. *What if Rob gets a call?* While it had not happened in four months, you never know.

Then, at 6:45 a.m., the phone rang. "Hello, Mr. Bellanich," the woman from Mayo Procurement said. "We are procuring a liver from someone who is brain-dead on life support with a good liver, the same blood type and size as you. The only thing is, you are the backup in case the primary patient tests positive for COVID. We need you to go to the third floor of the hospital by 8:30 a.m. to get your COVID test."

Our plans changed in a flash. We got up, threw a bag together "just in case," kissed the kids goodbye, and drove forty-five minutes to the almost empty parking lot at the Mayo Clinic, which looked extremely different in face of the pandemic.

The building felt lifeless with only a few people at the main entrance front desk and no one at all on the transplant floor. I went behind the former welcome desk where Bobbi always smiled checking people in. Instead, I found our hepatologist, Dr. Keaveny, barely recognizable in his mask. He directed us to another area where masked humans took us into a patient room. After a short wait, the nurse said that they could not do the rapid COVID test there; we'd have to go to the drive-through testing location behind the clinic.

So we returned to the car and followed signs to the testing unit in the huge parking lot, which looked like something out of a movie. Signs directed cars to small tents where people wearing masks and gloves were making hand gestures. After three checkpoints with people raising up signs to communicate and Rob putting his driver's license and Mayo number in the window, we drove to the actual testing tent where another woman came out, covered from head to toe in what looked like a beekeeper's gear. Rob finally rolled down his window. She took out a huge swab and put it way up both nostrils, which made Rob almost gag. "You do not want to go through that," he told me.

Rob asked me what my gut feeling was about the transplant, and I said I didn't think it would happen because anyone waiting for a liver would know to quarantine to avoid COVID. Unfortunately for us, I was right. Soon, we got the call that the primary patient was getting the liver, so we could go home.

While we were naturally disappointed, we were grateful the Mayo Clinic was still doing transplant surgeries, and someone sicker than Rob would be getting a good organ. I wondered who it was.

Facebook had been a good vehicle of expression for me, and with Rob's permission, I now began sharing his health struggle. I wrote frequent, detailed posts to update friends with both words and pictures, educating them about organ donation and transplantation in real time as I was educating myself. The response was quite overwhelming, which also gave me the confidence to continue documenting all these stories. Writing was both cathartic and gave me a purpose. I had another interview scheduled, which kept me going.

Lynn, whose story follows, was one of the first people Rob met in the Mayo support group. She gave him a small, smooth rock in the shape of a liver with the word "Courage" on it, which Rob carried in his pocket as a sign of hope.

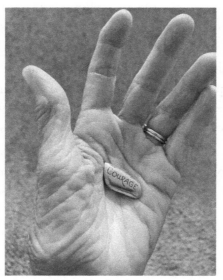

Lynn holding the "rock of courage" in
the shape of a liver

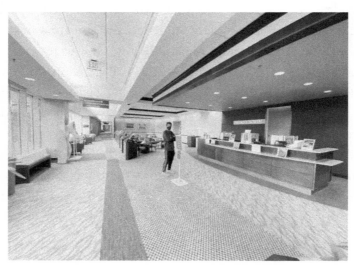

Rob standing in the empty Mayo Clinic floor

CHAPTER 12

Lynn: Secrets and Resentment

"I can't keep a secret," Lynn told me in our video conference. "If you want to keep something private, don't tell me. I just have to get it out." Her smile and spirit were infectious.

Lynn grew up in Montreal, Canada, and there were some secrets in her family revolving around health. Her mother had a cancerous lump removed from the roof of her mouth when Lynn was sixteen years old, but her father kept this from her, saying her mom went to the hospital for minor surgery. Five years later, the cancer returned, and major facial surgery was required. Afterward, the surgeon said, "I got as much as I could. I recommend not telling her to protect her." The decision to withhold this information caused tremendous resentment years later when Lynn's mother realized the truth. And after losing her mother in 1972, Lynn found that drinking alcohol was a good coping mechanism for her own anxiety and distress.

"Before I got sick, I was a very 'successful' (not) closet alcoholic," Lynn admitted. "I was never a falling-down drunk. Nobody ever knew, especially my husband, David. My parents were not drinkers. I didn't drink until college. Somewhere in my late twenties, I discovered that a beer could ease the anxiety attacks I was having after my mother died, and we were moving around with David's career."

By her late forties and fifties, Lynn realized she had to have a drink or two or three every night. Lunch was even better. "So, as they say in Alcoholics Anonymous (AA), I liked a drink, then alcohol liked me and wouldn't let me go!"

Hospitalized for depression in 1997, she quit drinking, but five years later she began again. Some time after that, taking prescription drugs along with alcohol, she saw a therapist who convinced her of the danger. "Slowly, I weaned off the pills and the booze. But then, I made a few deals with the devil and thought I could drink socially again. Secrecy and resentment. These have been big themes in my life," she said.

"Before my transplant, I led a 'normal' life. I had four children, volunteered, taught preschool after my youngest was born, ran two marathons, and played competitive bridge until two days before my liver failed on the streets of Boston—on March 29, 2014, the anniversary of my mother's death. This date is just as significant as my transplant, because I nearly died twice in the hospital—and I stopped drinking for good."

The previous fall, she and David were living in her family cottage in Quebec, and she had not been feeling well; she was unusually tired and had ferocious nose bleeds at times (which she later learned is a sign of liver failure).

"I knew I was an alcoholic. AA told me that years ago. But denial is not a river in Egypt," she said. "The day I collapsed, we had driven from Quebec to Boston to visit our daughter, Kate. My eyeballs were bright yellow, but for some reason, David never noticed. Kate did and said we were going immediately to the ER. Once we got there, I don't remember much more ... my memory went blank for ten whole days of my life."

She had slipped into a coma. Her son, Tyler, was getting on a plane to come from Australia when she apparently started to improve. Her husband never left the hospital the whole time. "One night, he noticed I was having a little trouble breathing so he went down to the nurse's desk, and the nurse said she would make a note in my chart and tell the doctor in the morning. 'No,' David said emphatically. 'I think you need to look now.' Sure enough, they called a code blue, and off I went to ICU. David saved my life," she declared.

When she came out of the coma, Lynn couldn't walk; she spent three weeks in the hospital and three more in rehab, learning how to walk again.

She and David went back to Canada, sold the cottage, and moved to Connecticut to be close to their oldest daughter, Ryann, and two hours from Boston and Massachusetts General Hospital (MGH). "They determined that my liver was in end-stage cirrhosis, told me not to drink for six months (like I ever would), find a therapist, and then they would consider me for a transplant," she said.

In December 2014, she was accepted into the MGH transplant program. She took a lot of meds and saw the hepatologist every three months. "I was on the list at MGH, but there was very little communication. No one told us to stay by the phone, and there was no support group. It was more like, 'You will probably live for a few good-enough years and then maybe receive a transplant.' I did not get a personal hopeful feeling."

In early 2016, Lynn was seeing an infectious disease doctor, who said bluntly, "What are you doing hanging around Boston? There are fewer livers here, and if you get sick, MGH might not be able to save you. Why aren't you considering the Mayo Clinic?"

Lynn came to Mayo in Jacksonville that April for evaluation and was thrilled to be accepted. She and David moved to Florida July 1— temporarily, they thought—to wait for a possible call. When they met with the pre-transplant social worker, Lynn asked her about a support group. Yes, they had a support group for transplant recipients and caregivers, meeting every Tuesday morning.

"At our first meeting, I introduced myself saying, 'Hi, I'm Lynn, and I am an alcoholic.' For some reason, I thought there would be other alcoholics there, but I was wrong. They were all talking about PSC, PBC, hep C, and it was Greek to us. Everyone in the group was welcoming, and I did not feel judged. I knew it was where I belonged. I still don't mind saying that I am an alcoholic because honesty helps me cope."

That summer, Lynn and David temporarily relocated to a condo on the beach. By September, feeling their wait was going to be much longer, they decided they would go home to Connecticut at the end of the month. "The average wait time at Mayo, we were told, was six months to a year, so they said if I wanted to go back to Connecticut for a while, I would just go on the 'inactive' list," Lynn said. "Fate had other plans."

September 10 was her birthday. "Three of our children came to visit since we had this condo on the beach," she recalled. "We had dinner reservations at a restaurant. At 8:30 p.m., my phone rang."

The screen showed "Mayo," so she went outside to take the call.

"Hello, are you Lynn?" a woman asked her.

"Yes," Lynn replied jokingly. "Are you calling to wish me happy birthday?"

"Yes! We have a liver for you."

"I was so shocked that I accidentally hung up the phone!" Lynn recalled. The phone rang again immediately, and David spoke to the caller, learning the hospital had a surgery time set up.

They got to the hospital by 9:30 p.m.; the transplant was scheduled for 2 a.m. with Dr. Burns. "The liver was on its way by airplane. I was probably a back-up recipient, but we never asked. It was a miracle," Lynn said.

"I can't talk about that night without tearing up. Why me? I feel like I died three years earlier on March 29, 2014, in Boston, but my mother was there watching over me, for sure. And to receive the call for the gift of a second chance at life on my own birthday—it just doesn't get any better than that, after only waiting two months."

Lynn found the Second Chance support group so helpful before, during, and invaluable after her transplant. "It was the main reason we decided to move permanently to Jacksonville," she said. "We have found a community of friends here just like me. We all speak the same language ... transplants!

"David as my caregiver was amazing," she added. "He has little patience with himself, gets irritated and 'vocal' if he can't tie his shoe properly, but for three weeks, he was almost saintlike! We recipients say that recovering, while painful, is easier than being a caregiver."

Although Lynn did not have the mood swings that some others described from medications post-transplant, she did have auditory hallucinations—mostly when she tried to sleep and would experience loud, jackhammer-type noises.

"As for recovery, many say six months before you are back to your old self. It wasn't like that for me. I just kind of dropped back into my old life, except without the alcohol and the secrecy. Now, I have nothing to hide, but I do admit to still having resentment that I could never drink socially like a 'proper lady,'" she commented. "Except for my never-ending gratitude that I was given a liver in order to live, I feel like 'me' again."

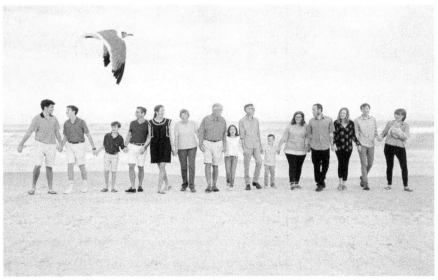

Lynn, David and their family

CHAPTER 13

Second Dry Run

April 7, 2020, St. Augustine

Three days after being turned down as the backup recipient, we got another call. Rob put the phone on speaker so I could hear.

"Hi, Captain Rob, it's Tommy from Procurement. We might have a liver for you, but there are some things you should know. It is a high-risk liver because it has hepatitis C."

"Okay," Rob said. "I know I agreed to accept a hep C liver, but what does that actually mean?"

"Well, after transplant the doctors would give you medication that is about 99 percent effective in eradicating the hep C."

"Is there anything else you can tell me about the donor?"

"Well, since it is high-risk, I can tell you that the donor died of a drug overdose. If you want to accept this offer, then you need to go to the ER at Mayo and get prepped for surgery."

Suddenly, we were getting ready to go again. We told the kids, and they got so excited that they started doing what they called "the liver dance," howling and jumping up and down in the condo.

We called our friends and family, drove to the hospital, then went to the transplant floor where Rob began testing to prep for surgery—including COVID testing again, EKG, blood work, and chest X-ray. First, Rob was given a "soft time" for surgery. We got on a video Zoom call with several of his transplant support group friends who were excited and giving him encouragement. Lynn was even joking about having to get an enema.

Soon, we were given a "hard time" for surgery at 8 p.m. It was looking promising. The timing would be ideal, I thought, because we could be back home before summer and the beginning of school.

At 7 p.m., an RN came into the room. "I'm sorry to tell you this," she said, "but when the surgeon looked at the liver, he was not happy with the way it looked."

"What does that mean?" I asked.

"The surgery has been called off. You are free to go home."

And just like that, it was over.

When I remembered this date was Passover, that suddenly had a dual meaning for us. On one hand, we all hoped that the coronavirus would "pass over" us just as the last plague passed over the Jews in the story of Exodus. In our case, Rob was once again "passed over" for a liver transplant. While we were devastated yet again, we had to trust that the doctors knew best.

This was the furthest Rob had gotten towards his transplant.

The irony was not lost on us that most of the world was frightened of having to go to a hospital due to COVID, and yet we were hoping to go back inside the Mayo Clinic for another chance. If it weren't for the hospital staff taking risks, we would not have had this opportunity.

I was told that the Mayo Clinic put the transplant program on hold for ten days until they could get COVID testing results in more quickly, since organs have a limited amount of time to be viable for transplant.

Rob had been living with PSC for eighteen years and on the national transplant waiting list for more than two years, with the last five months in Florida. We were so close, but all the stars had to align.

All over the country, sick people remained alone in hospital rooms due to COVID rules. The only surgery that allowed a loved one in the hospital room was a transplant because caregivers must learn what to do to help the patients afterwards. So I got to be there in the room with Rob while he was prepped for surgery and would be there through the entire process. I was grateful to be able to be by Rob's side.

After receiving the phone call from Tommy that day, I reached out to him to see if I could interview him for this book. I had no idea quite how complicated and thorough the process was. This turned out to be one of the most informative chapters.

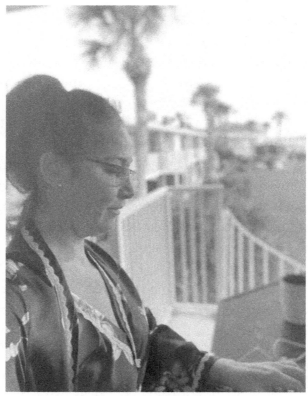

Lezlee writing on back deck of condo

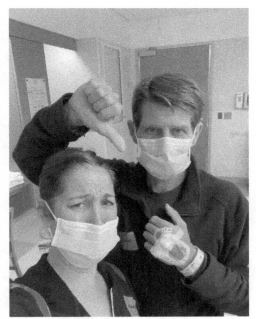

Rob and Lezlee finding out
the surgery was called off

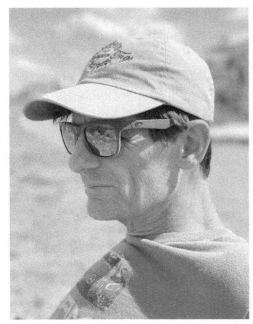

Rob getting thinner

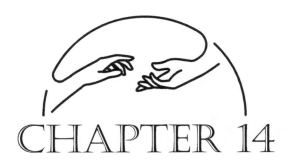

CHAPTER 14

Tommy: The 'Organ Traffic Controller'

If you ask Tommy Mulligan's eleven-year-old daughter, Brenna, what her father does for a living, she says, "My daddy gets people organs." And that is true. As the senior member of the Organ Procurement coordinator team at the Mayo Clinic Transplant Center in Jacksonville, Tommy is responsible for receiving and evaluating offers from organ procurement organizations (OPOs) when donor organs are available.

He works with Mayo transplant surgeons to match organs with patients on the waiting list and coordinates the retrieval of those organs from the designated hospitals where donors are on life support machines keeping their organs perfused and oxygenated. During his shift, he's the one who calls the patients eagerly waiting for an organ, gives them the basic information that he can legally share, obtains their acceptance, and tells them when to be at the hospital to prepare for surgery. He does all of this from his home office with three computer monitors and a headset.

Ten years ago, when he started this job at Mayo, there were only three coordinators, and now there are six. "We do a lot more than many other centers with our small staff, and if current trends continue, we will need more of us," Tommy said. He has seen the number of offers exponentially increase.

"My title at Mayo is a bit misleading because it's important to understand that there are two types of coordinators working together," he explained. "There are the organ procurement coordinators, called OPCs, who reach out to the donor family at the ICU, and the transplant coordinators—like our team at Mayo—working on behalf of the patients needing an organ."

Transplants are increasing in part because OPCs are better trained at approaching donor families to confirm their consent, as well as managing the donor's medical information to ensure the organs are suitable for transplant, Tommy has found. "On the transplant side, we are becoming more aggressive, and, thanks to improved medicine, vaccines, and advanced biomedical technology, we now can accept organs that we would have otherwise not been able to use."

The United States has fifty-eight federally designated organ procurement organizations, each with its own service area. Transplant centers work with a multitude of regional OPOs. In northern Florida, for example, the OPO is LifeQuest Organ Recovery Services. The organizations work to increase the number of registered donors by encouraging donor sign-ups and coordinate the donation process.

Because the U.S. has an "opt-in" system, meaning you must indicate whether you want to be an organ donor, first-person consent is checked off on a person's driver's license. Otherwise, the family must give consent at the critical time.

"If you die at home or at the scene of an accident and your heart stops, that's it. You could still be a tissue donor, but not an organ donor, because you must have blood flow and oxygen to the organs for them to remain viable," Tommy explained. "This is why the person must die in a hospital and be on a ventilator to keep the organs alive with enough time for proper testing so that organ offers can be made, accepted, and then transplant centers can procure the organs."

The OPCs are the people on the front lines who get the call from a hospital's intensive care unit notifying them of a patient who is legally brain-dead. The OPC travels to the hospital to make sure all the important tests have been done, speaks to the family during this delicate period, and uploads the medical information into the United Network for Organ Sharing (UNOS) computer system that is the vital link to the transplant centers. UNOS, a private, non-profit organization, manages our nation's Organ Procurement and Transplantation Network (OPTN) under contract with the federal government.

The main organs procured for transplant are heart, lung, liver, kidney, and pancreas. Kidneys, the most frequently needed, can stay viable outside the donor's body the longest—up to twenty-four hours; therefore, a patient can be on a waitlist farther from their home. Some organs and tissues can be donated by living donors, such as a kidney, bone marrow, or part of the liver or pancreas, but most transplants occur after the donor has died.

Born in 1968 in California, Tommy grew up in Mahopac, New York, and received a bachelor's degree in business at Bryant University in Rhode Island. After moving to Florida, he worked as a massage therapist and then in the restaurant business before entering the medical world. His then wife finished nursing school and suggested he, too, go into this field.

"I was always health-conscious, loved science and medicine, and was that nerd in school," Tommy described himself. "So, after I put her through school, she put me through nursing school at the University of Central Florida." He earned a critical-care scholarship, completed his accelerated nursing program in 2004, and began working on the cardiac floor at Florida Hospital in Orlando. He later went on to receive a master's degree in nursing education from Walden University.

"What got me interested in organ procurement was a Discovery Channel special I had seen before nursing school. I thought the field was so cool and felt, 'I would love to do that someday,'" he said. His chance came in 2006 when a position opened as an organ procurement coordinator at an OPO, TransLife. He was offered the job, which required a minimum commitment of three years as an OPC.

Every hospital has to call their local OPO when a patient is either about to have brain testing or has been declared brain-dead, or when the family is considering withdrawing their loved one from life support. "Let's say someone came in with a head injury from a car accident, and they are going to become brain-dead soon. That could become a five-hour process. If someone came in with a brain injury but was stable for days or weeks, an OPO does not get called until the end when it looks almost certain there is no chance for recovery," Tommy explained.

"The greatest myth that needs to be dispelled," he said, "is that if you are listed as a donor, we are going to swoop in and take your organs too quickly. No. First, we wait and see. Will the brain swelling go down if the patient had a head injury? After all other illnesses have been ruled out that could mask as brain death, two separate doctors come in and do the testing to make absolutely sure there is no chance of recovery. Brain death means that every single part of your brain is gone, including the brain stem—the most primitive form of the brain, which gives you the signal to initiate a breath." Once these tests are completed with no sign of brain function, the patient is declared legally dead.

"As a procurement coordinator," Tommy continued, "before we even get in the car and drive to that hospital, we are going to ask that bedside ICU nurse a lot of questions to understand the donor's medical history. Sometimes, after this conversation, a potential donor is ruled out—maybe for a simple reason that their blood pressure has dropped so there's not enough blood flow and oxygen to make organs suitable for transplant." This lends to the shortage of organ donors. Not everyone qualifies.

"When people list themselves as an organ donor on their license, the chances of them actually being a donor are very slim," he said.

According to the U.S. Government Information on Organ Donation and Transplantation, only three in 1,000 deaths occur in a way that allows for possible organ donation.

"Sometimes a family member cannot emotionally accept the situation and will not agree to donation," Tommy added, "and the OPC may find out why they are so opposed and convince them otherwise. It's important that the OPC gently talk to the family for a while with love and compassion before mentioning organ donation. It is usually not that the family is against donation, it is the fact that all of their choices, including their loved one, have been suddenly ripped from their life."

He went on, "It is confusing when someone walks in the ICU room and sees their son, daughter, husband, father, wife, or mother breathing with a ventilator and a monitor showing a heart rate, but then is told their loved one is dead with their organs only being kept alive by the machines. They don't realize that if those machines were turned off, the person would not take a breath on their own and eventually not have a heartbeat."

Often the concept of organ donation is a shock for the family because of an unexpected accident. "Their loved one may have left that morning, kissed and said goodbye, got in a car and had a freak accident or an altercation with someone, or perhaps tried to commit suicide. Now the family is being told that there is no hope of them coming back," Tommy said. "The family's end-of-life worries begin, and we are there in their face getting confirmation of consent for donation."

It's a tough balancing act, and he knows that the burnout rate for this job is usually eighteen months. "I was there three years to fulfill my commitment until I just couldn't take it anymore, especially when it came to children," Tommy said, choking with emotion.

An OPC puts all the data about each potential donor into the universal donor network system, instead of the old system of making many calls to transplant centers. This enables transplant coordinators at hospitals to evaluate the potential offer. A coordinator must know how the person died, gender, height, weight, age, blood type, lab values, organ function tests, X-rays, CT scans determining the size of the organ, and any disease or condition that could be transmitted to the recipient.

Tommy's daughter was born in the summer of 2008. In 2009, he took three kids to the operating room to be organ donors in one month. One of those children had died from a clear-cut case of neglect by that child's caregiver. "All judgment must be put aside for a parent who makes a poor decision," Tommy said. "A parent has the right to rescind consent for any reason for minor children. In that case, the tragedy happened, and there was nothing that could be done about it afterwards. That mother needed support, not judgment, to ensure the homes for her child's organs could be found, and another family's miracle could take place. Although I was part of the process of donation that would help other people, these experiences were too stressful. That was when I decided to go to the 'happier' side of the process."

He found that by becoming an organ transplant coordinator at Mayo Clinic. "To be a good transplant coordinator," he said, "you really need to have been on the other side as an OPC so you know exactly the time constraints and every question to ask."

There are many critical steps towards making an organ match, as Tommy explained. "Once we get an offer for a liver, for example, first, I look at where one of my Mayo Clinic transplant recipient patients is on that organ list. For livers, that is the MELD score, which correlates to mortality. I have a list generated each day of patients, for example, on the liver waiting list with their blood type, disease, height, weight, and an assigned surgical score from one to five, reflecting the likelihood that they'll have a relatively easy surgery based on their history and overall health. After looking this over, I call the appropriate surgeon to go over which person on the waiting list is appropriate."

Typically, the offers coincide with the distance from the donor, within 250, 500, 1,000, or even 1,500 miles. "The most common question is 'where are you on the list?' But there are so many factors that have to be taken into consideration at one time, and the list is always changing," Tommy said.

"Once we accept that offer, I call the matched recipient to go over the organ, offer information that I can share by law, and give them a soft timeline. Then, I call the operating room and the blood bank to figure out the timing of everything, including ground or air transportation to take the surgeon and assistant to the donor ICU to procure the organs.

"While we are coordinating all these details, we're still making sure the liver is good enough for transplant, sending out emails, making calls, and that is just for one organ. At the same time, I could have other offers for a right lung, a kidney, or a heart in a completely different hospital. This is why I have three computer monitors with multiple tabs open. One has my emails; the other is the schedule of who is on call, the current list of offers, details of the latest waitlist recipients in order of need (their disease, blood type, body weight, and so on). You could do all of this, have a backup recipient, and prep the recipient for surgery, but once the organ is in the hands of the surgeon, the doctor runs further tests on it. If there is even a hint of doubt, the surgery is called off, and the organ is not used."

Tommy explained some of the progressive changes that have been made in recent years. One example involves the "clock" of how long the organ can be viable once procured. The time needed to get organs out of the donor, travel time, and transplant surgery to put them into the recipient must be calculated in the total time. Clocks for hearts and lungs are usually within four hours; livers are eight to ten hours. There are now external biomedical devices that can test and prolong the viability of an organ outside the body (ex vivo).

He pointed out that UNOS has strict governing laws regarding donor and transplant. You can't buy your way to the top of the list or use any kind of personal connection to get yourself an organ. You can, however, relocate to another region of the country with lower median scores. Also, while a person can choose to donate certain organs to another person either as a living donor or after death, there can be absolutely no financial exchange between the parties.

When it comes to sharing donor information with recipients, there is a strict code of privacy to maintain anonymity. "We can't tell a recipient where the donor is from, their age, or race. One of the reasons is because people could judge it. If you are a forty-year-old who didn't take care of himself, you're a worse donor than a sixty-year-old who has been health conscious. Sometimes people are limited by what they think they know, and it is up to us to decide the best donor placement," Tommy said.

"Are we going to put a sixty-year-old kidney in a twenty-year-old person? No. But would we put it into a fifty-five-year-old person? On average, you're going to get ten years or more out of your new organ if you take good care of it. Also, you can get another transplant afterwards if you are still qualified. You can tell the recipient how the donor died, but without giving too many specific details, because with social media, people could search and find their donors, and we have to protect the donor families," he explained.

"If the donor's organ is considered high risk, then I am going to tell you why it is. High-risk could mean the donor has been incarcerated or potentially had anal or unprotected sex with multiple partners or engaged in risky behavior such as IV drug use—anything that the potential recipient needs to be aware of."

The transplant center also gets last-minute offers—for example, a kidney or liver may be offered after it has been removed from the donor's body. "Sometimes this might happen because when they go to take out the liver, for example, it is much larger than expected, and the doctors realize it is not going to fit in the intended recipient, so another home for it needs to be found quickly. Or, if the intended recipient is young, in their twenties, and the donor liver ends up having some fat or fibrosis, it becomes clear that it is better to transplant into an older person. The surgeons are always the ones who make the call as to who the recipient will be."

In many European and other countries, if you don't want to be a potential organ donor, you have to "opt-out" of the system; it is understood that you may be a donor unless otherwise indicated. And those who opt-out are placed at the bottom of waitlists if they ever need a transplant.

"Would it benefit the donor pool if we changed our policy from opt-in to opt-out? Probably," Tommy said. "But we are a country that focuses on individual rights so it would never work. Nobody in America wants to be told what they are supposed to do with any of their belongings, especially their body."

He emphasized that one of the best things you can do is to have a conversation with your family and loved ones about whether or not you or they want to be organ donors. "We spend most of our insurance money on end-of-life care because we hold on. I have noticed that sometimes the more religious a person is, the more they tend to hold on instead of letting go. Most of the major religions, however, are pro-donation. Both the Quran and the Torah say 'to save a life is to save humanity,'" he added.

"Organs are gifts," Tommy emphasized. "There are not a lot of good ones available compared to the needs of others, so you have to be very selective when offering them to a transplant patient, which is why there is a full evaluation process. Psychology, sociology, finance, pharmacy, support system, nutrition, and all department representatives have to agree that this person is deserving of taking a chance at being on the transplant list.

"Transplant is the only medical specialty where you are judged," he concluded, "because we have to know that you can and will take care of this gift when you receive it.

"Personally, this job has given me a real zest for life. We're not promised five more minutes. The reality is we never know what will happen. There is only so much control we have over the universe. When you realize and accept it, you try and live every day like it is your last. Love the people you love, and let go of the rest."

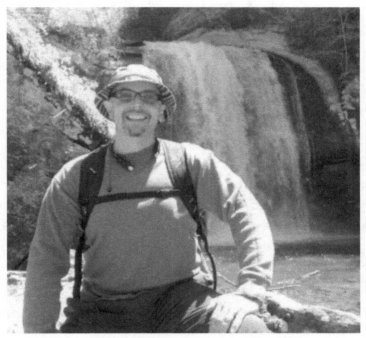

Tommy Mulligan, Organ Procurement Coordinator

CHAPTER 15

A Family Copes with the 'New Normal'

Late April 2020, St. Augustine

After being in our condo as a family for one whole month, this was our new normal, even if the kids were unhappy. If their school in Nyack had not been shut down for in-person learning because of the coronavirus, we would have just come down for spring break and gone home again. But instead, River and Skye were having to finish up their last quarter of school virtually with their laptop computers and an unstable internet connection.

From my perspective, this was miraculous because we were able to wait for Rob's transplant in a beautiful setting while being together. It didn't take long, however, to see the effect that the pandemic was having on the educational and emotional state of our teenager and pre-teen.

Our fifteen-year-old son did not embrace his new surroundings easily and began to shut down. His grades plummeted, and he began holing up in his dark room angry that his life had suddenly changed. Our daughter adjusted better, but she was only eleven. She missed her beloved guinea pig, Mishi. We had left so fast, but fortunately, friends had volunteered to take care of her pet.

While it was nice that the kids each had their own room in the condo, St. Augustine was not their home, and they never expected to stay there indefinitely. They were not only having to be isolated but

76

also in another part of the country. They missed their friends, and Rob felt terribly guilty. While he pushed himself to take us out on our tugboat, his fatigue made him irritable.

Financially, this was hurting us. Our yacht chartering business was at a complete standstill. We had charters booked, but not being able to operate, we encouraged our clients to reschedule. We were paying our mortgage in New York and renting the St. Augustine condo, while maintaining all the expenses for our dinner yacht without any income. Our health insurance company was not covering relocation or housing expenses, although from doing interviews with others, I learned that some insurance companies did cover relocation expenses for transplant patients.

Still, I felt fortunate. Mom left me a small cushion for "a rainy day," and it was pouring. Another transplant patient encouraged Rob to apply for disability benefits, and I applied for pandemic grants, unemployment insurance, loans, and everything I could think of to stay afloat. Not knowing how long we would be in Florida, we discussed renting out our home in Nyack for the summer. I knew we would be okay. We always landed on our feet. We had the sun and the sea. We had each other.

One week, as we were participating in the Tuesday support group meeting via Zoom, we heard a new voice. As soon as Ruth started talking, I knew she was a New Yorker with a powerful story.

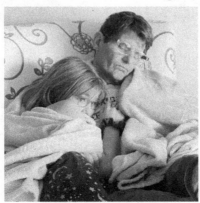

Rob resting with Skye

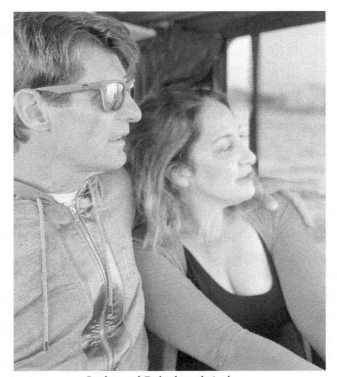

Lezlee and Rob aboard *Andiamo*

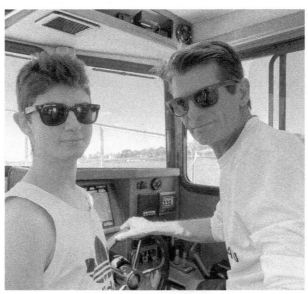

River and Rob steering

CHAPTER 16

Ruth: Even After Surviving Two Comas ... Still in Denial

"Ruth, how much alcohol do you drink a day?" the doctor asked Ruth after she passed out in her home one morning and was rushed by ambulance to the ER in Bayshore Long Island, New York. Doctors knew she had internal bleeding and needed a pint of blood immediately, but with her rare O-negative blood type, she had to wait until midnight because there was none to be found.

An endoscopy revealed the source of the bleeding: varices, or swollen veins, caused by liver disease. That's when the doctor assumed she was an alcoholic and pressed her to be honest. The truth was, neither Ruth nor her husband drank or had any alcohol in the house. Her brother-in-law, who was indeed an alcoholic, had been told his liver would regenerate if he stopped drinking, but Ruth, who was suddenly assumed to be an alcoholic, was soon told that only a liver transplant could cure her fatty liver disease.

Ruth, whose parents had come from Puerto Rico, was born in Brooklyn, New York. She studied accounting at Brooklyn College, and in 1976, at age twenty-one, she married her high school sweetheart, Wigberto, also from Puerto Rico. Wigberto (often called

Wig) operated his own barbershop before going to work for the State of New York as a custodian and later supervisor.

The couple had two children, Erica and Vanessa. Ruth had ample energy, and when her younger daughter was three years old, she returned to work to prove to her husband that she could indeed do it all—first working at a Sears Service Center and eventually as assistant sales manager at Paychex.

Her daughters grew up and got married, and the family traveled all over the country enjoying life. Other than having diabetes, controlled first through medication and then insulin shots, and high cholesterol controlled by medication, Ruth enjoyed good health, and she felt fine. She assumed that any fatigue she had was a result of having a fulltime job and simply getting older.

After learning in her late fifties that she had full-blown cirrhosis of the liver, she was referred to a specialist at Mount Sinai Hospital, who told her she could have a "good five years" before she needed a transplant. So she continued working, traveled to Europe, took care of her parents, and lived life to its fullest.

"Even though I knew I had liver disease," Ruth said, "for the next three years I was taking good care of myself, felt good, thought my liver would somehow regenerate on its own, and I would be fine. I wasn't worried about it. That was my attitude."

In December 2017, one of her co-workers noticed she began to "look a little yellow." Since she had turned sixty-two and was feeling more tired, vomiting more regularly, she decided it was time to retire. "Still, I didn't think it was my liver disease. I just chalked it up to doing too much," she recalled.

Travel and normal life continued the next year. A versatile musician, Wigberto often played at their church. Near Christmas, he was preparing for the church's holiday concert, but Ruth was too tired to attend. She felt like sleeping and could not wake up. Worried, her mother called Ruth's best friend, who came over, but Ruth suddenly did not recognize her friend. They drove to the church to get Wigberto, who knew that she was taking lactulose, used to reduce the amount of ammonia in the blood of liver disease patients; too much ammonia buildup causes confusion. They gave her more lactulose, and her head cleared up.

"We went to church Christmas Eve, and the next day, I made dinner at home for about twenty-five people," Ruth recalled. "After everyone left, I was exhausted and needed to lie down, and my feet were very swollen. Wig went to work and kept calling me, but I didn't answer. My parents were living upstairs, and when they came down, I was unresponsive." They called 911, and an ambulance took Ruth to Southside Hospital, where she stayed in a coma for five days. "Those days are out of my memory," she said.

"On the last day, December 30, I remember my daughter saying, 'Mom, if you can hear me, squeeze my hand.' I remember squeezing her hand, opening my eyes, and seeing so many people around me in that ICU room. I knew I was in a hospital, but I didn't know why. There must have been thirty family and friends there staring at me."

She came home a week later, extremely swollen, with so much water in her body that it was constricting her lungs. Ruth's doctor, Dr. Ahmad, at Mount Sinai wanted to see her immediately. "He took one look at me and admitted me, so I stayed in the hospital for another two weeks. They performed paracentesis, removing the fluid in my abdomen with a long, thin needle. That's one of the fun parts of liver disease, when you look ten months pregnant. My MELD score was about twenty-seven," she recalled.

"You will die in New York," Dr. Ahmad told her. "You have a rare blood type that is hard to match, and you are already going into encephalopathy from the ammonia building up." Both he and Ruth's gastroenterologist did their internship at Mayo Clinic in Rochester, and after conferring with each other, they convinced Ruth to go to the Jacksonville Mayo Clinic in February 2019. Both doctors called Mayo and had her records sent.

Thinking it would take months, Ruth was shocked when Mayo

Clinic called a few days later and scheduled her first evaluation for March 18. She learned that their health insurance through the State of New York fully covered both her transplant in another state and her travel expenses, including airfare, housing, and food for both the patient and the caregiver.

Ruth and Wigberto flew to Jacksonville and stayed at the renowned Gabriel House of Care, a nonprofit hospitality house that provides affordable, temporary lodging to hospital patients and caregivers coming to Jacksonville for organ transplants or cancer treatment. The Gabriel House of Care was conceived and funded by Jorge Bacardi, a double lung transplant recipient, and his wife, Leslie. The Bacardi gift to Mayo Clinic was an expression of their deep gratitude to their donor, Christopher, who Jorge called Gabriel after the heavenly archangel Gabriel. Located on the West Campus of Mayo Clinic, the house serves other nearby hospitals as well. It provides complimentary amenities such as yoga, art therapy, tai chi, and cooking classes, as well as ways to bond the guests for a family atmosphere.

"I loved staying at the Gabriel House," Ruth said, smiling, "because there were another thirty-nine families going through the same thing. We were not alone. We weren't stuck in a hotel room.

"I didn't have the Second Chance Support Group because I was so sick, but I did have the Gabriel House as my support group. There are no televisions or kitchens in the room, encouraging us to go downstairs and socialize with each other. Even now, there are about ten families who will pick up the phone and call me to see how I am doing. We are a family. "

Ruth spent three weeks getting evaluated for both liver and kidney transplants. Her kidney function was still fine, but liver disease affects kidney function, so that is part of the MELD score. To be listed for transplant, she needed to relocate to Florida, preferably not more than four hours from the hospital. So, in early April, the plan was that Ruth would stay with her daughter in Melbourne, Florida, three hours away, and Wigberto would go back to New York until she got a transplant, as he had to keep working.

"We are a religious family, and I have always had great faith believing that God works in mysterious ways. My husband kept telling me not to give up because God is good and would be my healer. I had friends and family constantly praying for me. This faith kept me steady. I refused to whine. I never said 'poor me' or 'why me?'" she said.

On the way home from a family outing after the weeks of Mayo evaluation, Ruth's daughter said she didn't look good and wanted to take her straight to Mayo. Ruth told her she was fine and went to bed.

"The next thing I knew, I woke up and had no idea where I was and scared out of my mind," she said. "Apparently, my husband heard me gurgling at 2 a.m., unresponsive, and he and my daughter took me to Holmes Regional Medical Center in Melbourne where I stayed in a coma for eight days. My ammonia levels had skyrocketed."

When she came out of the coma, she was transferred to Mayo Clinic for another week. "Even though I had just come out of a second coma, in my mind I still didn't think I was that sick. I knew I had liver disease, but for some reason, I still thought I would get better. It wasn't until two days before my transplant that I finally came to terms with the fact that I was indeed dying."

Getting out of the hospital on Mother's Day weekend, she returned to her daughter's home, where she planned to stay until receiving a transplant call from Mayo.

"On Monday, I knew, from having two comas, what the symptoms were. I told Erica I was not being stubborn anymore and to take me right away to the Mayo Clinic. We drove straight there, with my ammonia levels rising quickly. The bilirubin levels, which determine how jaundiced you get, had tripled," she recalled. By Tuesday, doctors said she was on a rollercoaster ride, and they were very concerned. She had diarrhea and indescribable pain with about forty pounds of fluid in her body.

"On Wednesday, one of the doctors told me the rollercoaster had gotten faster, and unfortunately there were no breaks to be found," Ruth told me. "I looked at him and asked if this was the time to call my friends and family to say goodbye. He shrugged his shoulders, looked like he was holding his emotions back, and walked out of the room."

That evening, Ruth sent up a special prayer. Her MELD score had risen to forty-three, considered the highest risk for liver transplant candidates. "God, I'm in your hands," she prayed. "It is your will, not mine. If you want to give me a liver and a kidney, I will be grateful, and I will praise your name until the day I die. But if you want to take me with you, I am physically, mentally, and emotionally done. I can't take this anymore. I am ready." Then, she went into a deep sleep, the first comfortable sleep she'd had in a long time.

"Two hours later, I woke up and someone was holding onto my arm, explaining he was about to draw twenty-five vials of blood. This seemed odd to me. The nurse came in and said, 'The bad news is we have to take a lot of blood. The good news is that we found a liver and a kidney for you!' I started screaming, 'Thank you, God. Thank you, God!'"

To find somebody her size with the rare RH O-negative blood type, where both the liver and kidney needed to match, was truly a miracle in Ruth's eyes. The kidney must be more of an exact match and it was. On May 17, 2019, at 2 a.m., Ruth got her transplants.

"Thank God, I did not have any complications. Even though I found out I was getting the organs on a Wednesday night, they were not procured right away and did not arrive at Mayo until 9 p.m. Thursday, a few hours before I had the surgery," she said. "When my husband walked into the hospital room the next morning, I was sitting up in the chair eating my breakfast. He could not believe it."

Expecting to be in the hospital for a month, according to her doctors in New York, she was shocked to be going to the Gabriel House only eight days later and on a plane to New York six and a half weeks later.

Today, Ruth feels like her old self. She usually walks three to four miles a day. After she got home in June, she found out that her mother was diagnosed with end-stage heart failure. Ruth took her to the hospital many times in the next three months.

"Instead of taking it easy, I was too busy taking care of my mother to sit back and worry about myself. Now I see that this was the best thing for me," she said. "The transplant to me meant that I had the opportunity to take care of my mom. God gave me another chance at life, and I had a purpose to make sure my mother was comfortable. I could not be more grateful for this second chance."

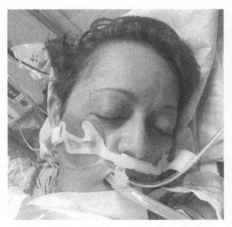

Ruth just after transplant surgery

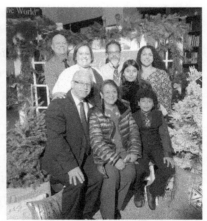

Ruth and her family

CHAPTER 17

Life and Death on May 4

May 2020, St. Augustine

May 4 will always be a day of duality. It was the date my mother was born in 1941 and the date she died in 2019 (her *yahrzeit*).

While I had lost close family members before, I never feared or had to face death like I did during my Mom's illness. She truly had "the happy gene," and her joy for life was infectious. She was timeless, and I could not imagine a world without her. Furthermore, in the last year of her life, it was the first time I had spent so much time in a hospital setting, listening to doctors, looking at monitors, and passing the time walking the corridors hoping for a miracle. Who knew it would prepare me for what was to come?

A year later, on May 4, 2020, we were in Florida, where we thought Rob had a better chance of getting a transplant. Rob and I both felt that something consequential would happen that day. Somehow, we believed that Mom's spirit would miraculously bring a liver match. Yet many people in the support group had told us that the call would come when we least expected it. We expected it, and it didn't come.

Instead, a completely different event occurred—a sudden family bereavement. We learned that my cousin's three-year-old son had tragically died from drowning. A precious toddler. I was shocked and incredibly saddened for the entire family, who lived two hours away in Ocala, Florida.

A disquieting thought also flashed before me. In an instant, someone's heartbreaking loss could save a stranger. But to approach a grieving family member, especially a parent, would be unthinkable. And yet, this was something Tommy from Procurement at Mayo described doing when he had worked for an organ procurement organization that approaches potential donors. I held my children a little longer that day.

Every day, every moment, every breath is so precious. None of us know how long we have. Some souls, like this beautiful toddler, come into this world for a brief period and make a big impact. Others stretch into longer periods of time. Who would be Rob's donor? To us, he or she would be a stranger. Their death would crush another while lifting our hope for renewed life.

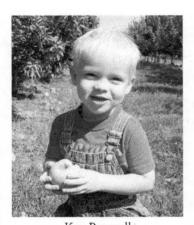

Ken Peterzell

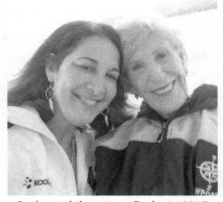

Lezlee with her mom, Becky in 2017

CHAPTER 18

Louis: The Ultimate Experimental Success Story

When transplant recipient Louis first shared a small bit of his story on one of the virtual support group meetings, I knew I needed to meet him. Since then, he has become a friend who checks in on me regularly, sending me uplifting texts like, "Hello, Lezlee, you have touched a lot of people in a very special way."

His frightening nightmare began in Orlando more than twenty years ago. "The results of your biopsy have come back, and you have a five-and-a-half-by-five-inch malignant tumor in your liver." These words from a cancer specialist shocked and scared Louis at forty-three years old.

At age nineteen, he had come alone from Nigeria to the United States to study mechanical engineering. He led a healthy lifestyle, ate well, exercised regularly, and had no reason to suspect anything unusual. In fact, for months prior to this news, when he complained of pain on his upper right abdomen, his doctor told him that he'd probably only pulled a muscle. Eventually, his doctor sent him to a specialist.

After a sonogram in 1997, Louis was diagnosed with a hepatocellular carcinoma. At that time, the word "cancer" sounded like a death sentence. Suddenly, he heard a loud voice in his head saying, "Don't worry, Louis. You will be fine."

Then, as if waking from a trance, he looked the doctor straight in the eye. "Doctor, I know what I have. Now you tell me, how am I going to be cured?"

"I'm sorry to tell you, Louis," the doctor responded, "but you may only have a week to live. My advice is to go home and get your affairs in order."

Louis said clearly, "Sir, I want you to tell me the best place money can buy to treat what I have." The doctor looked at him as though he was crazy, but Louis waited patiently while he called four hospitals—among them, the University of Pittsburgh Medical Center (UPMC).

"Well," the doctor began, "there are colleagues working on a new experimental treatment for cancer at University of Pittsburgh."

Before he could finish, Louis blurted out, "This is where I want to go."

"You know, your insurance is not going to pay for this because it's experimental," the specialist told him.

Looking back, Louis realized this might have stopped him, but something inside him compelled him to stand up. "I want you to pick up that phone and call my primary care doctor," he demanded. "You tell him what I have and where I want to be treated!" That was the beginning of his journey to surviving and thriving.

One of six children from a Catholic family in Kano, Nigeria, Louis had grown up in a home where the language spoken was English, as well as the local language, Igbo. His father owned a transportation and motor parts business and gas stations. His mother, a seamstress, designed and sold African clothing. Education was an expectation in their family; like many African youths, Louis went to college in America.

Accepted at Northeastern University in Boston, Massachusetts, he arrived there on Christmas Eve, 1974. "I was wearing a suit but did not have an overcoat yet," he recalled. "When my plane landed in Boston, I expected my uncle to pick me up, but he was not there. When I stepped out of the airport to look for a taxi, the blast of cold air was such a shocker! This was my first experience with icy winter weather." Later, Louis found the uncle had thought he was coming the next day.

When he graduated from Northeastern, Louis joined Stone and Webster, working in different parts of the country as a field engineer. He was often the only Black engineer on a power plant construction site. While on a project in Indiana, he was welcomed with open arms by the people even though the community was small and mainly white.

"Perhaps it was because I was from a foreign country," he pondered, "or perhaps it was because I was educated. But most people have always been nice to me. I believe if you look into people's eyes, they see who you are. I know there is racism in America, but I have always tried to understand the struggles and challenges of individuals, hoping peace will continue to bring everyone together."

In 1987, Louis went to work for EG&G Florida, a ground operation contractor at the Kennedy Space Center (KSC) near Orlando. He transferred to McDonnell Douglas (later merged with Boeing), which provided technical support for the KSC Space Station Program.

Louis married an African American woman in Boston in 1981, and they had a son, Christopher, the following year. Later, they adopted a little girl, Eucharia. After several years, the couple began to drift apart. "I stayed in the marriage for the children and because of my religious values," Louis said. "But after I lost both of my parents and was diagnosed with liver cancer, my wife filed for divorce in 1997."

For the next four years, while going through the divorce and losing close contact with his children, he flew back and forth every two weeks from Orlando to Pittsburgh for cancer treatments. When he'd first arrived at UPMC, he'd noticed most of the patients were wealthy. How else could they afford this experimental treatment? "Here I was, again, the only Black person. I just thanked God, knowing I was in the right place."

His initial treatments included gel foam and chemo embolization, a minimally invasive treatment intended to shrink the tumor. "After the first treatment, when I returned to Florida, I started running a high fever and was admitted to the hospital. The doctors in Orlando, however, did not understand what was happening. Remember, this was all experimental. They called doctors at UPMC, who said this was just a response to the treatment." When the fever broke, Louis soon was back at home.

Six months later, his tumor had shrunk by half. Doctors at UPMC performed a liver resection, removing fifty-one percent of the liver. The surgeons had been able to remove most of the tumor, but further testing showed tiny tumors along the resection line. Louis' journey continued.

"When we encounter devastating news," he reflected, "what often carries us through is our faith and our will to live." Doctors began a new type of outpatient radiation treatment, and Louis kept traveling to Pittsburgh every two weeks.

"I was blessed with living angels," he told me. "My Delta Airlines angels upgraded me to first class every time I flew. My gate agent angels would have my wheelchair ready for me when I got to the airport and when I got off the plane as I was so frail, I could barely stand up. The concierges at the hotel near the hospital treated me like a king. I felt support everywhere."

Finally, in 2000, three years after the first cancer specialist had told him he had a week to live, Louis' blood levels normalized, indicating he was cancer free. However, two years later, he learned the cancer treatments had been so harsh on his body that his liver was failing. Now he needed a transplant.

Living in Florida, it made more sense to get listed there with the shorter average wait time. His records were immediately transferred from UPMC to the Mayo Clinic, and he was put on the transplant list in the summer of 2002.

Many family members didn't think he would live much longer, so they were coming from all over the world to see him. One day, when cousins came to town, they headed for Disney World. "Mayo had given me a pager, and while we were on our way to the park, I got my first call for a liver transplant," he said. "I told the clinic where I was and that I'd take a cab back home and call from there. I told the Procurement coordinator that if I did not get back in time, please give the liver to someone else. When I got back home and called, they had given the liver to someone else. The way I looked at it, the other person needed it more than I did."

The second time he was called, it happened at 11:30 p.m. He reached out to three friends who had offered to help him, but each had an excuse. "Finally, I called my electrical engineering manager and friend, John, a wonderful white guy, who lived in Titusville," Louis said, smiling. "He didn't hesitate. We decided to meet at his house, which was on the way to Mayo." He managed the forty-five-minute drive to John's house, and his friend drove him to the hospital where he went through all the pre-surgery testing protocol.

The next morning, a nurse came in and said the surgery had been called off. The donor liver was not working properly. It was a "dry run," and Louis and John drove back in silence.

Then, while at work on August 31, he got another call. When he called his colleague, John responded, "C'mon, let's go!" And off they went. Louis had his liver transplant that same evening.

Four days later, however, his body had started rejecting the liver, and he had complications. "It's not like you can just go get another one," Louis joked. He stayed in the hospital almost two months while doctors tried to stabilize him. "Once again, no one thought I was going to live," he admitted. "Finally, they had to send me home, and once again, John drove me back to Orlando."

"I have had the most wonderful nurses in the world," Louis said.

"One nurse called me almost every day to check on me as I waited for my second transplant. I had to do my blood work at the lab near my house, and the test results were sent to Mayo. That nurse would read me the results by phone. She would cry as she was reading my numbers because they were so bad. I kept assuring her that I was not going anywhere."

Five months went by, and his next call for transplant came February 22, 2003. "And who do you think took me to the hospital?" Louis laughed. "My friend John. He told me to stay put and said, 'This time I'm coming to pick *you* up!'"

At the hospital, Louis was prepped for surgery. "As I was wheeled to the operating room for the second time," he recalled, "a nurse pointed at the liver surgeon who was preparing the organ and said, 'That is your new liver.' Looking at it quickly, I realized that I am probably one of the very few people who can say 'I have seen my liver.'"

Immediately after the surgery, an emergency developed— a small artery apparently was twisted, causing a stoppage in blood flow. Doctors needed permission from a family member in order to operate again. Miraculously, one of Louis's good friends happened to call from Boston to check on him. Asked whether he was family, the friend said yes—and to do whatever was needed. The surgeon quickly opened Louis up again, fixed the problem, and closed him up.

"When I woke up," Louis said, "it was like I had a different machine in my body. God had sent the best of the best to me. Even the president couldn't have had better treatment. I felt alive for the first time in a very long time. At night, my room became the nurses' station. Everybody gathered around me, so excited, saying I was a miracle. I had broken all the rules."

While the support group at Mayo Clinic at that time was smaller than it is today, it was a wonderful outlet for Louis, and he continues to participate in weekly Zoom meetings. Over the years, he has been a support for many people going through transplant.

In 2010, Louis took early retirement, having been advised by a co-worker that this would ensure that his health insurance premiums continued indefinitely at a fixed, lower rate.

Twenty-three years after a diagnosis of fatal liver cancer—and now having felt healthy for seventeen years after two liver transplants—Louis offered some simple words of wisdom. "I would like people to appreciate the moments they have and recognize how precious each moment truly is. Try to live life in a joyful, happy manner using every opportunity you have."

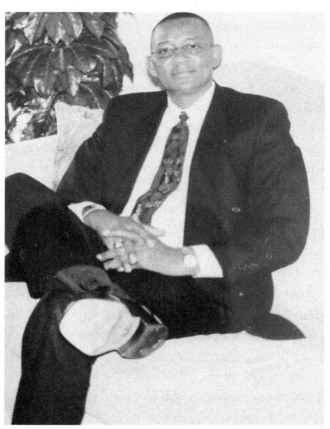

Louis

CHAPTER 19

This Waiting and Stress Became Unbearable

June 2020, St. Augustine

After three months living together in Florida, it was clear that this was not a normal situation. We were in a pandemic, displaced from our home many miles away, waiting for Rob to get a liver. We worried about contracting COVID and giving it to Rob, which would disqualify him from transplant, and we were unable to control the situation. We were four individuals at different ages and stages of life with different wants and needs. Ultimately, we were just a family, like every other, trying to get through this.

We had wanted to keep our children's lives as normal as possible in the relocation, but now that was impossible. There's an old saying, "You are only as happy as your least happy child." Our son, who had always been happy and relaxed, was angry.

As a ninth grader, just before we left New York, River had experienced having a girlfriend for the first time only to be separated from her. He barely ate, staying in his dark room lying on the bed staring at his computer. Every week, I got a call from the school telling me he was missing assignments and his grades plummeted. While some of his behavior was that of typical teenager, this situation had exacerbated it. Online learning was definitely not working for him. All he talked about was how much he wanted to go home.

Skye, too, hugged her stuffed animals and cried out for "Bebe," my mom, which broke my heart. She even talked about "wanting to go to heaven to be with her." Even though my daughter only had her grandmother for the first ten years of her life, their bond was forever. Skye waffled between little-girl-like behavior, calling me "Mommy" and craving affection, or pushing me away seeking independence. We embraced often, and I told her that Bebe would want us to live a long, happy life.

My children felt isolated. It didn't matter that there was a beach to explore, a bicycle to ride, or a boat to go out on. They refused to accept this as their temporary home. Unlike me, they could not see the beauty surrounding us.

Rob did not react well to the family stress. With his fatigue, he stretched out on the sofa sleeping most of the time, and he took the children's dissatisfaction personally. Any hard conversation with River, in particular, made his stomach hurt, causing him to reach for the heating pad. In the mornings, I would escape on the paddleboard when the bay was flat, looking for dolphins swirling up and down without warning.

As the family caregiver, I had to remain calm and positive in the face of our challenges. Falling apart was not an option. But I often felt like a failure watching River and Skye struggle and Rob so sick, worried the children would only remember him lying down all the time. I felt like I was failing at being patient and being a good wife and mother.

Working on this book during those months was a fulfilling diversion for me. It kept me going and gave me purpose. Interviewing other transplant patients, discovering the extremes some of them went through, and seeing them now thriving helped me keep everything in perspective. I knew it was a way to help others as well.

What stood out to me about Joe, this stocky, bald-headed man with a deep voice, was that when he spoke about his transplant with the various virtual support group patients, he would often spontaneously break into tears. While he blamed it on the medicine, he had a beautiful way of accepting his emotional eruptions as part of his new life.

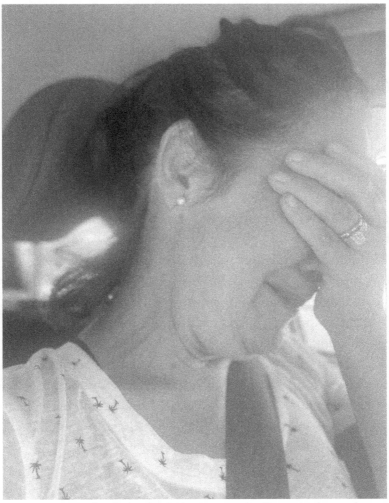

Lezlee dealing with the emotional rollercoaster

CHAPTER 20

Joe and Kathy: Overcoming the PTSD Emotional Rollercoaster

"**A** few months after my surgery, I went into what I now call PTSD after transplant," Joe told me with tears in his eyes. "That's when everything hits you at one time. It's a tough situation, and I think that's something that needs to be addressed more. It's not like you're losing your mind or anything, but all of a sudden, you wake up one morning, and the reality of life is right in front of you. Part of my emotional rollercoaster is from that, I'm sure, as well as the medication.

"It's a conflict where you feel so fortunate being on the other side of the fence, and then you look back at what you went through and what had to happen to get here. Now, if I hear a bang in the kitchen when Kathy is cooking, I jump eight feet. I can't take loud noises, even people talking. Large groups bother me. It's like I go into a panic, and the only thing I can compare it to is PTSD."

Joe received his liver transplant on March 10, 2019. For some reason, he and his wife, Kathy, who live in Naples, Florida, did not know about the Second Chance support group until the following year when it went virtual. This new platform opened up the group considerably, and for the first time, Joe participated and felt less alone—becoming part of a group of people like him who had gone through the transplant tunnel and survived.

Joe's health problems started in late 2010. After he suffered stomach pain, ulcers, countless endoscopies, transfusions, exhaustion, and mental confusion, Joe's gastroenterologist told him, "Joe, there's nothing more I can do for you here. If I were you, I would go to the Mayo Clinic."

He was accepted in the Mayo transplant program in 2013, and his health journey continued with more MRIs and other testing until he was diagnosed with non-alcoholic liver cirrhosis. For the next few years, he regularly made the five-and-a-half-hour drive from Naples to the Mayo Clinic in Jacksonville for ongoing care. After the appointments, he and his wife stayed with a relative in Jacksonville who happened to be a Mayo nurse.

"My MELD score never went over fifteen all those years, so I was not placed on the liver transplant list until 2018 and then finally transplanted the following year," he explained.

In our video interview a year after his transplant, Joe—a six-foot-tall man weighing 300 pounds—could barely get through a sentence without tearing up from emotions. He said he used to be a stoic, type A personality, but now he sees himself as more forgiving and laid-back.

"I barely made it," he told me. "Right before my transplant, my MELD jumped from seventeen to twenty-nine in three days. It was low for many, many years, but it did not reflect how sick I was, and I know I should have had the transplant much sooner. It wasn't until the cancer hit my liver that my MELD score shot up. I ended up with two malignant tumors in my liver, which were wiped out by radiated pellets. When this happens, you are radioactive for thirty to forty-five days, so transplants cannot take place. I also had a blood clot in my artery, so I had two strikes against me," he said.

"When they removed my liver, they found two other hidden tumors and realized that the blood clot was much larger than they thought. Thank God they were unable to detect them on the latest MRO. Otherwise, it would have been too late, they would not have done the transplant, and I would have run out of time."

Joe, whose father had been in the Air Force, signed up for the Navy in 1969 after high school, but he was turned down because his liver enzymes were high on a routine blood test. Joe felt perfectly healthy and appealed his case to Walter Reed Hospital, as many people his size have high enzyme counts.

The Army accepted him, and after completing the Reserved Officer Training Corps (ROTC) program at Inter-American University in Puerto Rico in the early 1970s, he did his basic training at Ft. Knox, Kentucky. "In those days, you went where they needed bodies. You didn't have a choice," he recalled. "They needed bodies to go into armor, which was tanks. From there, I was waiting to get orders to go to Vietnam as a tank commander. But that never happened because the war ended, and they had more bodies than they knew what to do with."

Joe moved to New Jersey and began teaching for five years. That's where he met Kathy, also a teacher. Later, they moved to Puerto Rico for him to go to law school at the Inter-American University. "I got to study both the Spanish and English system of law there, and I was trained in both civil law and common law," he said.

Because he lived in so many different countries as a boy, he had a knack for languages and could understand Spanish, Italian, French, and Arabic. His mother spoke Spanish and made sure her four children were bi-lingual, so he is most comfortable reading, writing, and speaking in this language. He and Kathy went on to have four children, two of them born in Puerto Rico.

Joe became in-house counsel for a manufacturing company in New Jersey, and when the children were in high school, the family settled in Naples to be near his parents. The company had offices in Miami, so he would split his weekdays in both cities. Life was good. Life was normal. Until it wasn't.

"When I started to get sick, I became dependent on Kathy for so many things. It was a slow and steady decline of not being able to walk, drive, or do much of anything," he recalled. "I was cold all the time and slept twelve to fourteen hours during the day. With bleeding in my stool, my hemoglobin counts kept crashing to about six, which for a guy my size is really low. They kept giving me transfusions to get it up, then it would come crashing down again. Also, I was turning into a space cadet. I could not count backwards from 200 because the ammonia was building up in my brain, causing encephalopathy. I felt like I had just run a marathon, so exhausted all the time. I was worried about doing something wrong and getting disbarred because I could not concentrate, so I quit working."

The family is Catholic, and Joe had to have last rites done four times by his priest, three of those while he was in the hospital different times. He was thankful that his doctor in Naples had taken good notes, which Mayo was able to use in diagnosing him. "Mayo worked directly with Dr. Phillips for various procedures like banding the polyps in my esophagus to choke the blood supply so they fell off," Joe said. "This stopped the bleeding in my stool."

"At the beginning of March, we were sitting waiting to go in to see the transplant team at Mayo," Kathy interjected. "Mike, the social worker, came out into the waiting room and could see how much Joe had deteriorated. He came over to give him a hug. When they called Joe's name, Mike came and sat with us for moral support. That's why we have such a special feeling for him; he showed what the people at Mayo were like. We went home on that Monday, and we got the call that Saturday. Dr. Perry, a five-foot-four-inch-tall woman, had just done three transplants in a row. She was amazing."

After the surgery, Joe's heart rate was high. "Some people go into atrial fibrillation after transplant," he said. "After tests, they determined my heart was in A-flutter, and I had an ablation just a few weeks ago."

"Shortly after Joe's transplant," Kathy added, "he just had a light sheet over him because his internal temperature was regulated. He looked immediately so much better. The staff at Mayo were our guardian angels. They are all incredible, going above and beyond. Joe could not walk into any of the departments at Mayo without someone saying, 'Hey, Joe! How are you doing?'"

"I have written my generic thank-you letter to the donor family but have not heard anything," Joe said. "All we know is that the donor came from the West Coast. I would love to meet the family and thank them. Maybe I will try again. I'm here because of Kathy," Joe whispered, choking up. "This woman has done stuff for me that—" He couldn't finish.

"You know, I never looked at it that way, and I told him that," Kathy said. "The day I said, 'I do" in front of the priest and committed to 'in sickness and in health,' those were the words I meant. We've had so many good times. This is just a little bump in the road."

"Has the romance come back?" I asked jokingly.

Both of them nodded a clear *yes* in response.

"We've been married forty-six years," said Joe. "We have four children and eight grandchildren. I fight through this for my family, especially to be there for my grandkids. When they tell you it's a new lease on life, they're not exaggerating. It's a long road, but it's worth it."

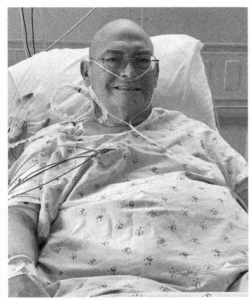

Joe in hospital post-transplant

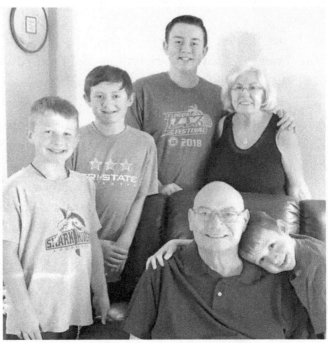

Joe and Kathy with their grandchildren

CHAPTER 21

Fourth of July Without Fireworks

July 2020, St. Augustine

There were no planned fireworks this year because cities and towns did not want to encourage crowd gatherings. July 4 is a celebration of our country's freedom, but none of us felt free. Breathing the same air inside or closer than six feet apart outside was dangerous.

When we left New York, we felt safer in Florida because there were fewer cases. By July, everything had reversed. Yet the response in Florida was different. No one wore masks outside unless they were in a crowded area, but everyone wore them in stores. I did all the grocery shopping and wiped everything down before putting it away. Rob could barely walk a few feet without getting winded. Still, his MELD score was only nineteen. How could this be?

We worried that if Rob tested positive for COVID when a liver transplant call came, doctors would not transplant him; if I tested positive, I could not be his caregiver. Still, I believed it was important to get out and breathe the fresh air. To preserve my peace of mind, I often rode my bicycle over the Bridge of Lions towards the historic downtown and residential section. As I made local friends, they knew our story, and many of them prayed for us. Having grown up in the South, I enjoyed the slower pace, though the summer Florida heat was debilitating.

While our environment was serene, we were in the middle of a perfect storm of challenges. Besides a complete halt to our seasonal business, we had a couple renting our Nyack house with continual questions—but mostly, Rob needed a liver transplant before developing sepsis or even bile duct cancer. It was a race against time.

When the New York governor loosened some of the restrictions, I was able to book a few small charters aboard the *Royal Princess* relying on our loyal New York crew to carry them out. Our charter business had survived 9/11, but this pause was much worse. The bills kept pouring in while the debt kept growing. The rules kept changing while the inactivity kept dragging on. And every day, Rob grew weaker, more emaciated with his skin and eyes a darker yellow. His spirit was beginning to fade.

As spring turned into summer without an expected call, I began developing a little thing called faith; faith that everything would be okay even if it wasn't in that moment, faith that we would indeed go through the next tunnel and get to the other side, and faith in a higher power watching over us. If I jumped too far ahead, I became anxious. But if I took things one step at a time, life felt manageable. When I focused on projects that made me feel engaged and purposeful, I felt productive. We were hoping for the best, preparing for the worst, and adjusting to our strange circumstances.

We were also juggling different "what if?" decisions such as: What if Rob didn't get transplanted by the end of the summer? Should we register the kids for school in Florida? That felt like implementing a death sentence to them, and my gut told me not to.

River got his Florida learner's permit so that he could practice driving, which was a highlight. Rob took him to the Florida Department of Motor Vehicles where he watched his son say "yes" when they asked if he wanted to be an organ donor. This brought tears to Rob's eyes.

Should we bring the *Royal Princess* down to Jacksonville and try to charter it in a new market? That seemed like an overwhelming amount of work. Rob felt it would do better in Florida, and someone would more likely purchase the vessel if it was there. I did not think we needed to relocate the whole business for a buyer to make an offer.

My husband shuffled around the condo like a zombie, hunched over, worried, with a pained look on his face. Our Second Chance support group friends kept encouraging us, assuring that Rob would have a rebirth after transplant. Maybe he, too, was developing mental haziness and confusion due to liver disease. For someone who was never afraid to take control of the wheel, he was losing control over his life.

At 9 p.m. on July 4, Rob, Skye, and I went out to our docked tugboat at the condo pier, and suddenly, all around us we saw fireworks. There must have been fifteen amazing, colorful displays exploding and lighting up the sky above the water and on land, thanks to local residents and boaters celebrating. Maybe it was a sign. When we least expected it, our own fireworks show would happen.

One support group member, Alicia, reached out to me as a mother when I mentioned how important it was early on to keep my children's lives as normal as possible. She, too, felt this way about her daughter during her transplant and understood the ache of being pulled as a parent wanting the best for your child.

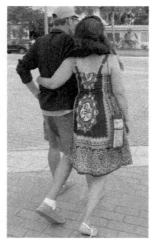

Fourth of July without fireworks

106

CHAPTER 22

Alicia: The Never-Ending Itch

Imagine your whole body itching twenty-four hours a day from the inside out, and there is nothing you can do to stop it. Still, you can't help scratching yourself with hairbrushes or utensils, using creams, taking hot showers, or doing anything you can think of to relieve the itch. That's what Alicia endured sporadically since she was only twenty-four years old.

In 1995, Alicia was diagnosed with primary biliary cholangitis (PBC), a progressive liver disease that destroys the bile ducts inside the liver. PBC is similar to primary sclerosing cholangitis, PSC—Rob's diagnosis, which affects the bile ducts both inside and outside the liver and is more common in men. More than ninety percent of patients who have PBC are women. Itching, also known as pruritus, is associated more with PBC but often occurs with PSC patients as well. Three years before Alicia's liver transplant on October 14, 2014, her itching was constant, relentless, and unbearable.

"It was a nightmare," Alicia recounted. "I took every possible drug early on to control it. Later, I took part in an experimental procedure called plasmapheresis at the Mayo Clinic, where they filtered my blood through a port, which gave me relief for twelve weeks. Then, as my disease progressed, the relief time shortened.

The nerves that cause itching are different from pain receptors. It's a feeling I can barely describe. I don't wish this on my worst enemy."

The condition was so bad that her liver specialist at Mayo Clinic went before the regional UNOS Board and, because her quality of life was so poor, argued for exception points to be added to Alicia's MELD score, which was only nine at the time. She was awarded more points, bringing the score to twenty-two when she was transplanted.

Born in Richmond, Virginia, Alicia grew up in the small town of Winchester, Virginia. "Dad was a forester and worked for the State of Virginia and then a paper company, going out and marking the timber to be cut down leaving enough trees so the forest could keep flourishing," she said proudly. "Mom was an office manager who also served as a state legislator for twenty years in the Virginia House of Delegates."

As a child, Alicia had missed a fair amount of school because of viruses and rheumatological problems with joint pains in her hands and feet. She graduated from Dowell J. Howard Technical School and became a licensed practical nurse, working for twenty years in Virginia facilities including an urgent care center. Her husband, Darryl, recently retired from his career as a Verizon Fios tech.

"I met Darryl when I was eighteen years old and he was twenty-six. He was driving by in the park, and I thought he was cute so I yelled at him," she told me, laughing. "He stopped, and my friend and I went for a ride with him. Pretty brave. We were married a year later, in 1990."

Only four years into their marriage, Alicia became fatigued and started to have strange itching for no reason. "I had an appointment with my ob-gyn because I wanted to get pregnant and wondered why it wasn't happening. She said she would run some lab work to make sure my body was ready to have a baby. My liver functions came back whacko. My alkaline phosphatase was eight times what it should have been. She told me there was something majorly wrong with my liver, so the baby thing went out the window," Alicia recalled.

"At first, a doctor considered it was my gallbladder or maybe a few stones. After exploratory surgery, the doctor did a liver biopsy. The results came back as primary biliary cirrhosis, which has four stages. At stage one, my liver was inflamed from the bile ducts. Of course, when you are itching constantly, it's not very romantic."

Alicia was sent to a local gastroenterologist, who prescribed medication. Wanting a second opinion, she went out to the Mayo Clinic in Rochester to see a hepatologist. "I had such confidence in the Mayo doctor that every year or every other year for the next seventeen years, I flew out there to be evaluated. I was prescribed many different medications for my itching. When one medication would wear off, I was prescribed another."

When her doctor in Rochester retired in 2010, Alicia began traveling to Jacksonville's Mayo Clinic every year. "Luckily, our PPO insurance allowed me to go anywhere for treatment," she said. "I did not want to be transplanted at such a young age as long as my disease was manageable." With PBC, patients usually have to get a transplant seventeen to twenty years after being diagnosed. Alicia was right on schedule.

Her daughter, Amanda, was born in 1997 and after her delivery, Alicia had some bleeding complications. With advice from her doctors, she decided to have tubal ligation a week later. "It was not an easy decision for a twenty-six-year-old to have her tubes tied," Alicia confessed. "I still think it was the best decision, and I don't have any regrets. I have a beautiful daughter, and I'm very blessed."

At age two, Amanda was diagnosed with juvenile diabetes. "That was probably one of the saddest days of my life because I knew as a nurse that this was a lifelong problem," Alicia recalled. She homeschooled her daughter until third grade, then found a private school where Alicia could be the school nurse and be with her. For high school, they returned to homeschooling. "That worked out because that was the time frame I got really sick, so she could come to Jacksonville, bring her work, and be with me," Alicia said. "She is an adult now, and I just want her to be happy and take care of herself from this disease."

In 2013, Alicia was diagnosed and almost died from complications of yet another autoimmune disease, lupus. After her 24/7 itching became so unbearable that she was unable to sleep, she was finally put on the liver transplant list in Florida in April 2014 even though her husband and daughter were in Virginia.

"Being separated from my family was the hardest thing I have ever done in my life," she recalled. "My husband and teenage daughter were still living in Virginia because he had to keep working and we wanted to minimize drastic changes in Amanda's life. They both were able to visit every month because Darryl could take family medical leave to see me. I'm so glad I was able to have my mother with me, or I would not have been able to do this. I was truly thinking that I would never get the call and had emotions all over the place. Also, I knew that if I was to live, someone else had to die, and this weighed heavily on my mind."

Alicia's mother was available to be her caregiver because, in the primary election, she had lost her seat in the state legislature, a shocking outcome because she was such a longtime member. "If you don't think that's God's plan," Alicia said, "then I don't know what else is because I couldn't have moved to Florida on my own financially or without my parents' support through this ordeal." Her father had leukemia, but he traveled back and forth from Virginia to Florida.

"While I was waiting for my liver, I found the Second Chance Support Group, and this was the changing point for my wait. They assured me that it would happen, and they were living proof of the whole process," Alicia said.

Her Christian faith has always been helpful to her. "In August, I was called by the Procurement nurse at 3 a.m. asking if I was willing to take a high-risk liver," she said. "This means they don't have a lot of information about the donor, and it could be risky for certain diseases. I prayed hard for the donor family, accepted the risky liver, went to the ER, and then to the transplant floor. They took a ton of lab samples and told me I had a hard time for surgery at 7 p.m. But at 7:30 p.m., a nurse came to tell me that the liver was not viable. I was very disappointed but again prayed for the family and went home feeling defeated."

She wanted to go back to Virginia because she was so homesick for her family. Each time Darryl and Amanda left after their monthly visit, she cried and counted down the days until their next visit.

Then, on October 13, her daughter called her from Virginia, sounding incoherent. "This call happened to be during our Second Chance Support Group. I knew right away that she was in trouble, so I called 911 and made sure they could get in the house to take her to the hospital. Then, I called my husband, who was an hour away at work, and he met her at the ER. She was put in ICU with ketoacidosis, which is extremely dangerous for diabetics. I went back into the support group very upset and told them I had to go home immediately. Between the group and my husband, they convinced me to stay in Florida and not come home. Reluctantly, I stayed while Darryl was with Amanda in the hospital, assuring me he had everything under control and that her sugar was normalizing," Alicia said.

"I'm sure glad I stayed because the next day, October 14, at 3 a.m., I received my second call from the Procurement nurse, and I received my gift of life at 10:30 a.m.

"When I woke up after surgery, I realized I had no more itching! There were a few postoperative complications including a twisted bowel and pneumonia resulting in an extended stay of nineteen days at the Mayo Clinic. Then, I continued on outpatient IV antibiotics upon discharge and started the recovery process— about ten weeks— and was able to return to Virginia by Christmas 2014."

Alicia's parents were both with her during her transplant, but her father died six months later. "His passing broke my heart," she whispered.

"After my rebirth, I was able to watch my daughter graduate, celebrate my twenty-fifth wedding anniversary, soon-to-be thirtieth, and start enjoying life again. I did acquire the cytomegalovirus from my donor and struggled from it for two years, but it finally resolved.

"I am five years out, and my liver is doing great. My whole family lives in Jacksonville now, as Mom stayed here. We are living the good life!"

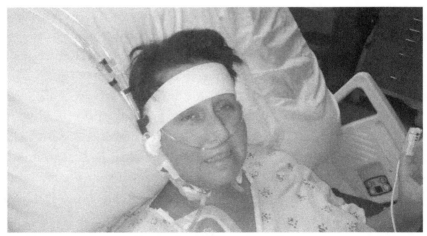

Alicia in hospital post-transplant

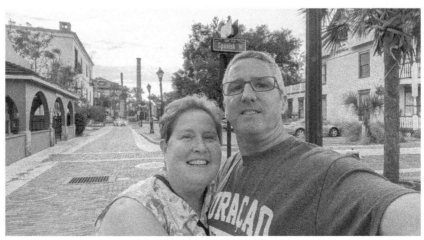

Alicia and her husband Darryl

CHAPTER 23

The Gary and Barry Show: Two Brothers' Transplant Journeys

During the first support group meeting I attended in 2019, there were two men who resembled each other sitting side by side. After our introductions, it became apparent that they were brothers, and they shared an astonishing story.

What are the chances that Gary and his younger brother, Barry, would both have liver diseases leading to liver transplants—done by the same surgeon at the same hospital eight months apart? For Gary, an analytical, computer-programming, self-described "nerd" who takes things as they come, it was simply a problem that needed to be solved. For Barry, a creative soul who looks at life beyond the surface, it was a surreal experience that "happened for a reason."

While their personalities are different, they grew up together and have remained close, bonding through their sense of humor and shared life history. Both share a Midwestern, straightforward way of speaking. Gary was born December 17, 1957, in Lincoln, Nebraska. "Dad wanted a tax deduction," he blurted with a grin. "So Barry was born by a scheduled C section on December 31, 1959." Barry laughed and agreed.

"Dad was outgoing and never met a stranger," Barry described. "I am more like him, but I temper it down."

"I am more laid-back like Mom," said Gary. She was a registered nurse and always healthy until she developed Parkinson's disease late in life. Their father had various jobs, including being a mental health technician at a state hospital, and he became a registered nurse at age sixty.

In fact, their dad went to the same nursing school where Barry had studied a few years earlier. At the time, nursing was changing, and more men went into the profession, traditionally dominated by women. "We were a rare breed," Barry joked.

"We had our spats as kids," he laughed, "but Gary was a good big brother. We played accordion together as children. Not much drama in our family."

When the boys were ages eleven and thirteen, the family moved to their mother's hometown, Jacksonville, Florida, which was a tough transition for boys of that age. Barry started playing bluegrass music on a banjo as a teenager, later learning the guitar, mandolin, fiddle, and electric bass, and playing in folk, acoustic, and jazz bands.

Gary graduated from the University of North Florida with a degree in computer science and began working in information technology. "Barry's the klutz, and I'm the genius," he laughed.

"Yes." Barry nodded. "That is true."

Both still live in Jacksonville, relatively near each other. Gary has remained happily single, and Barry married twice; he and his wife, Annette, have been married almost thirty years.

Barry has four children and four grandchildren. He walked away from nursing in 1986 and became a civilian calibration technician at the Mayport Naval Station.

For fun, Gary still works with computers. "That's my life," he smiled. "I build computers and program them. Barry and I don't get together that often, but as he said, we'd have the usual good conversation of 'How ya doin?' 'Fine.'"

Barry was diagnosed with liver disease before his older brother, but his transplant occurred after Gary's. Barry's health had always been good, but in 2010 a routine blood work test showed unusually elevated liver enzymes. His then primary doctor did not think a liver biopsy was necessary. Instead, Barry tried dieting and lost forty pounds; his liver counts went back down but then began to creep up again. "The train was already running along," he explained.

"My wife wanted me to switch primary doctors so I did. In the fall of 2016, the new doctor referred me to the Mayo Clinic, and once I went in, they didn't play around. They were very serious and thorough."

After testing, Barry was diagnosed with non-alcoholic steatohepatitis (NASH), the liver manifestation of a metabolic disorder, which is the most severe form of non-alcoholic fatty liver disease. The symptoms are often silent and difficult to diagnose. As a result, NASH patients can remain unaware of their condition until late stages of the disease.

"Mayo determined that I had stage four cirrhosis, which was shocking," Barry said. "Looking back, I was tired, but I didn't think it was that bad. In July 2017, we went to Disney, and I began to have swelling with blotches on my skin. When I went to see Dr. Keaveny at the Mayo Clinic, he informed me that they were putting me on the transplant list probably sooner than later. The word 'transplant' was frightening."

That December, Barry had his first "dry run." After all the preliminary recipient tests were done at the hospital, the doctor came in before surgery to say that the liver that had been procured was not a good one, and the surgery was called off. He had a MELD score of twenty-six, which he thinks had risen due to having had the flu recently. A few weeks later, it went down.

"The whole time that Barry was going through his diagnosis, I didn't think anything was wrong with me," Gary chimed in. "I was just concerned for Barry. My ordeal was fast. Everything was going along hunky-dory, and then, *bam*! My liver started shutting down."

Gary had never had any significant health problems. "During the summer of 2016, when I was fifty-nine, I noticed my legs and abdomen began to swell," Gary recalled. "This is called ascites. Basically, your liver becomes like a rock so the fluid can't go through it, and fluid builds up in your body. If I look back, a year before the transplant, I did have signs that something was wrong. Once I had a paper cut, and it continued to bleed without clotting. One of the symptoms of liver failure is the inability to clot. The summer before, I had dry, itchy skin. I hadn't seen a doctor in about fifteen years because I was never sick. Maybe if I hadn't neglected my health, I would have caught this a lot sooner because the numbers would have shown up on any lab test. I just never had my blood work drawn."

Gary's case was strange because doctors did not have a true diagnosis of this liver trouble, so it was called "cryptogenic," meaning unknown. They knew what it was not: It wasn't hepatitis A, B, or C, or alcohol-related. It was autoimmune-related, a disorder that did run in his family. By November 2016, Gary's liver was in full cirrhosis.

"Barry's wife wanted me to go to Mayo right away," he recounted. "But I went to a gastroenterologist first who couldn't figure out what was wrong, so he sent me to Mayo. At first, I thought it was only a referral, but the transplant coordinator scheduled me for an evaluation. Transplant? I was surprised. But after all the tests were done in early 2017, it was clear I needed a transplant so I was listed in March." He waited eight weeks, then got the call from Mayo, and was transplanted on May 1, 2017.

For Barry, being his brother's caregiver through his liver transplant was literally a preview of what he would experience the following year. He and Annette sat in on a lot of the classes with Gary and met him at the hospital on the night of the transplant.

Gary takes things as they come. He was not apprehensive. "People seem to work themselves up into an anxiety about this sort of thing," he admitted. "But I didn't have that. That's not my personality type. I think I take after my Aunt Dena, who was calmly sitting on her front lawn with one shoe off after her house burned down," he laughed. "Nothing flustered her. The Mayo Clinic explained everything to me so I knew what to expect and felt confident."

While Gary was in the hospital, he met another transplant patient, Jerry, at a nutrition meeting. Jerry asked him if he knew about the Second Chance Support Group. Neither of them had gone yet to a meeting, but after Jerry mentioned it, Gary thought it was a good idea. One week, he had some appointments on Tuesday and went downstairs to the meeting room. Since Gary worked during the day, it was hard for him to get to the meetings, but he went to some and enjoyed them.

Later on, both Gary and Jerry had some rejection issues with their new livers. When Hurricane Irma hit Jacksonville in September 2017, the two were locked in the Mayo Clinic for several days together with other transplant patients during the storm and got to know each other.

"I was receiving an infusion at the time," Gary said matter-of-factly. "Normally, it's a two-day thing, but I couldn't go home because of the high winds. All the nurses had to stay there overnight, and we stayed as well. It was an unusual, surreal experience." He grinned at the memory.

"Over the course of three years, I've had several bouts of rejection. You go in, get your labs, and if it warrants it, they give you a biopsy to look at your tissue. I think I may have had a record number of ten biopsies at Mayo. After the transplant, your nerves are severed around that area, so it doesn't hurt as much," Gary laughed.

Barry got his final call January 10, 2018, from a nice guy explaining what to do and where to go. "I told my wife it was like when a child is born or your wedding day. There's been so much build-up, you almost get to a point where you're just going along for the ride, and you'd like, at some point, to take a breath and be present in the moment. But they were so good at guiding me through every step of the process. It's a big deal. My wife was my caregiver, and Gary was a support in all kinds of ways," he said.

"Gary has always been there whenever I have needed him for anything. When I got ill, he helped me with no hesitation. He is a very giving guy and a man of few words but big actions. He's introverted but has a great sarcasm. Like when I asked him what he wanted for New Year's dinner, he said with a straight face, '*Not* liver and onions!'"

"When I was visiting Barry on the transplant floor," Gary recalled, "all the same nurses were there that took care of me. He was walking down the hall doing his exercises, and I was walking with him, and everyone was doing a double-take," he laughed.

The brothers tried to figure out how they both could have had their paths lead to the same point. Their diet and lifestyle were similar. They thought it was a genetic predisposition to liver disease. Now when they get together, they pull out their matching pill packs and take their meds at the same time.

The pandemic of 2020 didn't change Gary's work life much, except that he began doing it from home instead of his office. He does recognize the need to be more careful. But as he said, "They drill being precautionary into you at Mayo—like staying away from large crowds and washing your food under hot water for three minutes—but I don't go to the store that often."

Barry had a much more emotional reaction after his transplant. "I was very thankful," he said. "I'm a little more introspective. I look at it this way—we happen to live in Jacksonville near the world-renowned Mayo Clinic. Gary was ill. I was here. I was able to take off and take care of him. Then, he was able to take care of us. There's a greater source of events in our lives. I firmly believe that there is a reason that things happen to people, particularly after an event like this."

Barry's wife wrote a letter to the donor family. "In her letter, she said that they were praying for a miracle for their loved one to live, and we are praying on our end. There is a greater connection between people than we realize." Barry suddenly got choked up.

Does Gary believe there's a greater thing going on? No, and he's not apologetic about it, simply acknowledging that everyone deals with things in a different way. To Gary, it happened, it was an experience, it was dealt with, and he is at peace with himself because he sees the world differently. But he thinks it is important that people hear all types of stories because not everyone has a history of health problems or reacts to having a transplant in the same way.

For Barry, with his more spiritual nature, every day is different. He is on a different journey.

But they love and accept each other fully for who they are. Two brothers. Two transplants with two different perspectives, both recipients sharing a deep, heartfelt love.

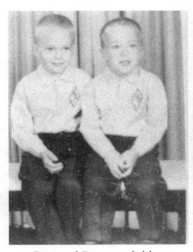

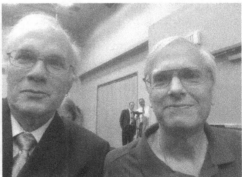

Barry and Gary as adults

Gary and Barry as children

CHAPTER 24

Looking to Friends for Strength and Hope

August 2020, St. Augustine

As we sat on the deck at sunset overlooking the water one evening, I could hear the anger and desperation in Rob's voice when he said, "Why, when I never drank alcohol or took any drugs, do I have this ticking bomb inside me?"

Something had set him off a few nights prior, and he'd stormed into the living room announcing that he wanted me to take the kids back to New York. A day later, he said that he felt like throwing in the towel and going back home to wait until his MELD score was higher.

Looking back later, he told my uncle Roy about his feelings during that difficult time when he'd been waiting so long. "I couldn't see the beauty around us. I was numb. Here we were trying to figure out our finances in the middle of this pandemic that shut down our yacht chartering business, which was our main source of income. Our children were displaced from their home. Our son was unhappy, missed his new girlfriend, and barely completed his online schoolwork, so I felt terrible putting my family through this.

"By the end of July, it was too stressful for me, and in a fit of anger, I lost it yelling at my family to go back home, and I would stick it out on my own. But Lezlee remained calm and wasn't going to let me do that, so they stayed."

Around his fifty-sixth birthday on August 23, he began to feel even more despondent. "I realized that my dad had died of liver disease at fifty-five years old, and I had made it a year past him," he explained. "One of the reasons I joined the Navy after high school was because I was so down at seventeen years old after he died, and I needed discipline. So, on my birthday, I kept thinking, 'How much time do I have? Another three months? Six months? Will my kids lose their father like I lost mine?' It just kept sticking in my head. The uncertainty was so difficult and I was losing faith."

For him, the frustration was severe. "What was going through my head," Rob later told Roy, "was 'I can't fix it,' and I am one who loves to fix things. I could not control this thing that was deteriorating my body, no matter what I did."

While Rob was struggling with the issues, I had been warned about some of the hazards many months ago by a friend I'd met through a PSC online support group. Kim had told me that things were "going to get really bad." Her husband had suffered with the same disease as Rob and had a liver transplant from a living donor a few years ago.

In my interview with our friend Louis, he'd talked about the "living angels" that were all around him when he was sick. We, too, had living angels.

Kim became one for me. Although we've never met in person, I would text or call her anytime with questions. She was the one who had convinced me to pack my bags in March and get on the next flight to Jacksonville. She knew that the sicker Rob got, the more he would need me. She was right. Also, the local friends we made—especially Callie, Lou, Carol, Greg, Melissa, Tommy, and neighbors in the Salt Run complex—were there for us. And I felt the support from family and friends like never before.

Rob's living angels were especially the pre- and post-transplant friends he made in the support group who gave him constant encouragement. "Don't lose hope, Rob," they would tell him. "Your time is coming. We just know it. And when it does, you are going to feel whole again."

Our social worker, Mike, also provided vital support. "Rob, let me remind you that you got called twice since being here," he said. "I can't promise when you will get called again, but your chances are much greater here than in New York. If you leave, you will be inactive. I know it is hard, but you have to hang on."

We needed our living angels. One day, we hoped to be angels to others.

Rob bonded with support group member John over their shared interest in nautical affairs. He and his wife, Trink, with her wide smile, were very welcoming to Rob when he was a new member of the group attending the in-person Second Chance meetings.

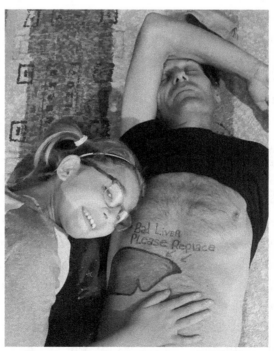

Skye draws a picture of a liver on her daddy

CHAPTER 25

John and Jennifer: A Niece Becomes Her Uncle's Kidney Donor

"I feel as though I won the lottery," John said with eyes wide open as we began this video conference with him, his wife, Trink, and his niece, Jennifer.

"And I am blessed that I was your winning ticket," Jennifer answered, smiling.

Originally from Michigan, John moved to Richmond, Virginia, with his family at age twelve. He and Trink met at the University of Michigan, dated in his final semester, then went their separate ways. Trink became a teacher, and John went into the offshore oil business in California.

One day, when he went back to the Ann Arbor campus for a fraternity alumni meeting, one of his frat brothers asked, "Whatever happened to that girl you dated?" John had no idea, but he called the sorority house in the middle of the night, waking up a student to ask about Trink. He learned that she had graduated and was living in West Covina, California, not far from Los Angeles, where John lived. Unfortunately, they had parted on cold terms.

It took John several months to get up the courage to surprise Trink with a visit, only to leave his business card as she was not at home. He smiled in recollection. "She read me the riot act about how arrogant it was to do that," he said. "It took me another three or four months to convince her to go out with me, just to have a margarita and talk about old times. We finally got back together and, within a year, were married."

It was 1969, with the military draft in full swing. Hoping for a critical-skills deferment, John found a job building commercial ships in Newport News, Virginia. He and Trink lived there several years and then moved back to Michigan, where John earned his master's in business administration.

"Our son, John, was born just a few months after Jen's birth in 1971, and they spent a lot of time together as babies," he says. He had grown up with two brothers, and Jennifer, his niece by marriage, was the first baby girl in his life. There was a special bond between them.

John and Trink went on to have a daughter, Lisa. As John was in the shipping business, they lived in port cities around the world. In 1991, a company he'd worked for received a contract from Saudi Arabia to clean up oil spills left from Saddam Hussein's invasion of Kuwait. The Saudis did not want the oil to wash ashore and clog up their desalination plants, and John was hired to oversee the cleanup. Since it was temporary, he went alone, and the family stayed in Philadelphia.

"When you got within 100 miles of Kuwait," John recalled, "the sky looked like it was midnight. The oil fires were so bad they turned the entire landscape black, and we were ingesting all that oil in the weeks we were living there." He paused. "That is the only place, I reason, where I could possibly have been infected with toxins that might later have been the cause of my bladder and kidney problems."

His niece, Jen, received her nursing degree from the University of Michigan, where she also met her husband, Kiyoshi. When the couple moved west, Jen worked at California Pacific Medical Center in San

Francisco, where she often found herself taking care of post-operative patients who'd had heart, liver, pancreas, or kidney transplants.

"It was my favorite job," Jen said. "I gained a pretty in-depth knowledge of the transplant experience. In my time there, I only met one kidney donor. I saw transplant recipients and I witnessed at least one heart transplant. I have both amazing and sad recollections from those days in the ICU," she admitted.

"For the most part, transplant is an incredible gift. You see patients going from being on dialysis to having a new, perfectly functioning kidney. And with liver transplants, patients go into surgery desperately ill. After surgery, the transformation that occurs is like a resurrection. Some patients, especially those with heart problems, are lying in a bed in the ICU, ready for a transplant, just waiting for someone to die. Many of them struggle with this concept even after they have received a transplant. With kidneys, there is another option. People who are alive can opt to donate because we all have two kidneys."

At the time, Jen did not envision herself personally going through the organ transplant process. "I'm sure at some point I must have thought, 'If I ever had the opportunity, I would do this,'" she said. "And, Lord knows, as soon as I got my driver's license, I indicated I wanted to be an organ donor. That's a no-brainer to me, and it surprises me that so many people do not fill out their organ donor card."

Jen and Kiyoshi always remained close to John and Trink, who frequently visited them. From California, Jen, her husband, and two children moved to Poughkeepsie, New York.

John and Trink retired in 2006 to Jacksonville, fifteen minutes from the Mayo Clinic. Was it coincidence or luck? Although not an overly religious person, John, nevertheless, believes that someone up there guided them to this location for a reason.

In retirement, he began having medical problems, and knowing Jen's nursing experience, he would call her sometimes to talk about issues with his atrial fibrillation, an irregular heart rate that can increase risk of stroke or heart failure. At a family reunion, after John had some cardiac complaints, Jen checked his pulse and told him to go the hospital. He was having a fast abnormal heart rate that could have been life-threatening.

On one occasion, John had to undergo emergency surgery in Jacksonville because his colon burst and it was leaking into his abdomen. Jen, who was working at Vassar Brothers Hospital in Poughkeepsie, immediately flew down to be with him when John's daughter called her.

"I had just completed a twelve-hour overnight shift," Jen said. "My cousin, Lisa, said her dad was in surgery for a perforated colon, so that morning when I went home, I caught a flight to Jacksonville. I knew the situation was serious. I arrived in time to be there when he came out of the ICU, and Trink and I took turns staying with him. I didn't think anything of it. My kids were in elementary school, and my supportive husband knows that when it's someone you love and you need to go, you just go and take care of things."

Several years later, John was diagnosed with bladder cancer. "My kidney function continued to deteriorate even after my bladder was removed in 2014," he said. "I was admitted into Baptist South Hospital with a urinary tract infection, informed that my kidneys had failed, and told I needed to go on dialysis immediately." He remained on dialysis three times a week for three years.

"When I started to investigate a transplant," John continued, "I called Mayo Clinic, and the first thing they asked was how tall I was I and how much I weighed. I was six feet tall and weighed 350 pounds. My BMI calculation was forty-six, which is considered obese. Mayo would not take me. I looked into transplant at the University of Florida in Gainesville and went through the evaluation process. They gave me the same BMI speech and told me I had to lose weight beforehand."

He decided to have gastric bypass surgery at Baptist. After losing 100 pounds, he pursued the Mayo Clinic again. "This time when

I called and told them my BMI was now at thirty-four, they said, 'Come on in!' They welcomed me with open arms, and that started my Mayo love affair," he said, smiling.

"Through all of these medical problems my uncle had been having, he would call me, and we would keep in touch," Jen recalled. "When my grandfather, Trink's father, passed away, we had a chance to meet up at the memorial service. We talked about his health struggles. He mentioned pursuing transplant, and right away, I told him that I would be willing to donate. He didn't have to ask me."

"I had never expected such a selfless act," John exclaimed. "Yet from Jenny's point of view, it was a 'natural' thing for her to do."

"At first," Jen said, "I thought, 'What are the chances I would be a match for him?' We are not blood-related. Yet when I had my blood work drawn in Poughkeepsie and had it sent down to Mayo, it indicated I was a match! The next step was a complete health evaluation. Once I got to the Mayo Clinic, I met with the surgeon, Dr. David Lee, and we clicked right away. He, too, had studied at University of Michigan."

She was impressed with Mayo's entire evaluation process. "They were so thorough, not only in assessing me physically, but also in presenting me with possible scenarios: What if my uncle was noncompliant post-operatively, would I have regrets? Would that challenge our relationship, and how would I handle it? They probed deeply to ascertain that there would be no negative consequences to me," she said.

"I understood that if one day I myself developed kidney problems, having kept my second kidney would be of no help. If one of the two kidneys in our body stops functioning, the other one does not simply take over. This is not the way our renal system works. However, even with just one kidney, if I kept myself healthy, I would not be compromised in any way. When the news came that I was a match, I said, 'Let's do it!' The level of minute detail that Mayo goes through in their evaluation process is exceedingly thorough. This is why their success rate is so good."

"The history with kidney transplants is that sometimes you wait five or six years for a kidney, and I was already three years in," John said. "I thought I'd be okay waiting, and then, out of the blue, Jenny said that she wanted to do this. I couldn't believe my good fortune or what magical hold I had over her because I didn't ever expect this. I didn't want her to do this. I didn't feel I deserved this, and it was the most selfless thing that anyone has ever done."

Jen's mom, a retired nurse, came down to be with her for the transplant in June 2017. "I spent one night in the hospital and was in Jacksonville for a week before going back to my family. I really didn't think about myself at that point," Jen said. "I was more concerned that everything was going to be successful for Uncle John, knowing his history of previous surgeries."

As is usually the case, John's health insurance paid for the testing and surgery for both donor and recipient.

A last-minute hiccup occurred the day before the scheduled surgery. John had already had a procedure creating a urostomy, an artificial opening for urine to leave the body, when his bladder was removed. Dr. Lee, originally wanting to insert the new kidney where the urostomy was located, ordered a CT scan to determine how and where to place the kidney with enough space and gravity to provide correct flow to the urostomy. As some doubt remained, the transplant process was altered.

"The new process," John explained, "was to have me brought into the operating room, open me up to see if there was enough space, and then, if acceptable, temporarily close my open wound, bring Jen into the OR, remove her kidney, move her to recovery, and finally, reopen my wound to accomplish the transplant. After consultation, that was the procedure that the surgeons followed. From start to finish, it took more than eighteen hours."

As a side note, Jen commented, "I asked the circulating nurse to say, 'Go Blue!" to Dr. Lee when my kidney was being handed to him in the sterile bowl, since it was going from one University of Michigan grad to another UM grad, then being inserted by a third UM grad. The OR team went one step better and played the UM fight song, 'Hail to the Victors'!"

"Since that monumental event, I have spoken to Jen many times about the fact that I need to take care of her kidney," John said. "I don't want to ever feel like I have fallen down on my end of the bargain."

His wife suggested they go to the Second Chance Support Group to see what it was like. "I am not a gushy person most of the time, and I didn't care to relive the whole thing. But somehow, when we went, a page turned, and it became very clear to me how much benefit this support group offers. First of all, there is a lot of intelligence in the room, and it is interesting to hear all the experiences other people have gone through," he said.

"The thing that keeps me going to the support group is seeing a new person come into the room. They have that 'deer in the headlights' look. They are frightened beyond belief about what they are about to enter into, not knowing if they will be accepted by the hospital, or if they are physically capable of having it done. Is this a pipe dream? Is this a wish that will never be accomplished? Will they go through all of the prep only to have someone tell them no?

"To see these newcomers enter the room, listen to the rest of the group, then offer comfort to try and calm that person's fears, walking them back from the edge ... to me, that is the most important help we provide. The group says, 'Hey, you're right. It is a major surgery, but this procedure is a proven, well-established technique, and you shouldn't be afraid of pursuing this because it will alter the rest of your life.'"

His heartfelt closing line brought our conference call to an end. But first, I admitted to him that our time waiting for a liver was beginning to feel like a pipe dream. Rob and I could not help but question whether it would ever happen. "Well, once you're through it all," John reassured me, "you're gonna look back and see this time as shorter than it felt in real time. The outcome will be so rewarding that you will know, looking back on it, that it was worth going through, whatever it took."

Thank you, John.

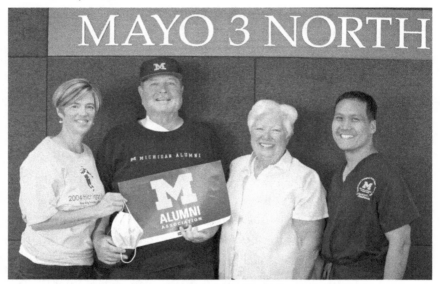

Jennifer, John, Trink, and Dr. David Lee, July 2017

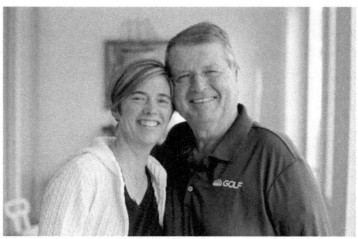

Jen and John together

CHAPTER 26

Outrage Leads to Action

August 2020, St. Augustine

My Aunt Dale often quotes the Serenity Prayer: "God, grant me the serenity to accept the things I cannot change, the courage to change the things I can, and the wisdom to know the difference."

Life was throwing its share of crap at us. I needed to figure out what I could possibly change to affect the outcome of our delicate situation.

The first challenge was making sure our small business health insurance plan would be renewed September 1 without question. We had paid high premiums on time all these years. We had chosen a plan that would give us the most freedom to go to an out-of-state hospital covered within the network. In essence, it boiled down to paperwork. We had to make sure that our company still fell within the legal definition of "small business." The health insurance options in the United States are so complicated that without a third party to explain it, it is overwhelming. With the help of our insurance broker, Laurel, and longtime accountant, Gary, we figured it out, but we certainly did not need that level of stress at this time.

The next dilemma was realizing that Rob was stuck in something we called "MELD Score Purgatory." His relatively low score, nineteen, was working against him. Even though he was clearly much sicker than when he first relocated, he remained on a lower priority on the waitlist, risking life-threatening complications.

After delving into policies of UNOS, I learned that a new policy had been enacted in February 2020, which changed the liver allocation system. While the intention was to make available livers more accessible in regions of the country like New York by changing certain rules, it inevitably made the MELD score matter more.

When liver transplant patients have their blood drawn, the MELD scores are calculated based on both their liver and kidney functions. Often, those patients with PSC have high liver counts, but unless they are experiencing fluid in the belly, their kidney scores remain lower, keeping their total score in a medium range. It suddenly dawned on me that Rob's MELD score did not reflect how sick he was.

When we went to see his hepatologist, Dr. Keaveny, he explained that as recently as a year prior, doctors could more easily make the argument to regional boards at UNOS to grant PSC patients exception points, which would raise their chances of being offered a liver. But currently it was far more restrictive. The national policy also changed to limit the possibility of PSC patients receiving exception points if they were hospitalized twice in three months with sepsis or developed cancer. This made no sense to me. Caregivers like me often become activists pretty quickly.

Once I realized the double whammy of what was keeping Rob and all patients with PSC or PBC from getting transplanted before severe complications occur, the more outraged I became.

"So, you are telling me that even though my husband is rapidly wasting away with murky-colored skin, yellow eyes, and little energy, he doesn't qualify for exception points?"

"That is correct," Dr. Keaveny said.

"Sir, I have a question. Do you think the MELD score is a fair assessment of how sick all patients with liver disease are?"

"My personal opinion," he responded, "is that the MELD score is not a perfect system, and, yes, it is indeed stacked against people with PSC."

I felt a hot sensation around my neck. "Well, do you think I have any chance of trying to change policy within UNOS to give exception points to people with PSC or PBC?" I asked him.

After a slight pause, he looked at me and said, "Why not? The squeaky wheel gets the oil." Right then, I decided to be that squeaky wheel.

———•———

When I started this book, I wanted to write about our journey through my husband's liver transplant, along with amazing and inspiring stories from other transplant patients. I set up video interview sessions, each lasting one to two hours.

After each story, I was shocked to hear how far the body could be pushed to the brink of death before a transplant. When we were in New York, we knew the chances that Rob might have to get deathly ill before receiving his precious gift. We also knew it is much riskier to be transplanted after being sick in a hospital from organ failure, sepsis, cancer, or being in a coma. From everything we read, saw, and heard, we thought it would be about three to six months before Rob would get his transplant in Florida, along with the fact that Mayo Clinic has a stellar reputation.

But the hospital cannot control when a liver becomes available or who is where on the waitlist.

It wasn't until I started interviewing so many people and studying the information on the United Network of Organ Sharing (UNOS) website that I began to understand the whole process of how a donor organ gets from the hospital where the patient dies to the recipient on the waitlist. In a nutshell, I learned that knowledge is power. Had Rob been transplanted quickly, I would not have looked more carefully into the national guidelines and learned how their recent policy expanded the liver allocation process.

To clarify again, UNOS is the private, non-profit organization that serves as the nation's organ transplant system—the Organ Procurement and Transplantation Network (OPTN)—under contract with the federal government. UNOS manages the national transplant waiting list matching donors to recipients according to policies developed by the community and approved by the OPTN Board of Directors.

UNOS divides areas of the country into regions. In the past, if a donor died in a certain region, that liver would go to the nearest transplant center because livers can only survive twelve hours outside the body. But in February 2020, a new policy called "Acuity Circles" went into effect. Now, livers would be offered to the sickest people in the transplant centers with the highest MELD scores within a larger radius—150, 250, and 500 nautical miles.

The goal of UNOS is to improve the equitable allocation of livers (and other organs) for transplantation for patients across the country on the waitlist. Unfortunately, the new policy put even more emphasis on higher MELD scores.

The public can submit comments, pro and con, to UNOS prior to policies being enacted, but I could not find objections about the acuity circles change on the public comments section of the website. Why was that? Who was reaching out to the transplant community asking for their input? Why weren't patients investigating the policies that were affecting their very survival? Why weren't more people participating? Perhaps because patients were not aware that they have a voice. In an effort to push harder for Rob, I took it upon myself to change that. And quickly.

On August 4, 2020, I started a petition on change.org entitled "Exception Points on MELD Scores for PSC and PBC Liver Transplant Patients." I explained the basic transplant terms and described our story as an example. The petition asked UNOS for exception points on MELD scores of transplant patients with PSC and PBC, who are often sicker than their scores indicate. I did not know what the reaction would be.

In one month after sharing the petition on my Facebook page along with every social media group related to the issue that I could find, over 6,000 people signed it. Soon, we had over 9,000 signatures.

More importantly, when I spoke to the PR director at UNOS, Lisa Schaffner, she explained the importance of public comment as a metric for policy changes. In only a few weeks after the petition, nearly forty people with PSC or PBC left public comments on the UNOS website, which everyone on the National Liver Review Board reads. Patients told their stories of agony waiting longer for transplant, and family members expressed their horror when their loved one was too sick for transplant or died after developing cancer or sepsis. We were only one family of thousands who felt the same way.

Then, after the floodgates opened, the PR director asked us to join a video conference with people who work at UNOS, where Rob and I got a chance to speak directly with them on behalf of PSC and PBC patients. After we pleaded our case, the team assured us that UNOS was listening. And they were.

I found myself communicating with so many people from around the country who have reached out in various ways, through the petition, Facebook pages, UNOS site, and other media.

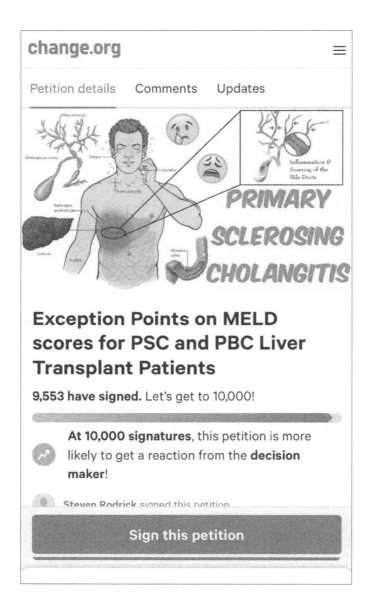

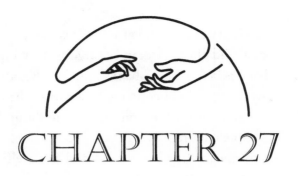

CHAPTER 27

Cici: Not One, Not Two, But Three Transplants

Transplant patient Jerry, an early supporter of my book, told me that I absolutely needed to interview Cici, who was at Mayo Clinic during his ordeal and who had kept up the spirits of others. I am so glad I did.

What did Cici learn from having a kidney and three liver transplants over the course of six years? Mostly, she learned about patience and forgiveness. How else could she have endured this? "It's not my time," she kept telling herself after waiting and waiting. "God has a plan. The right liver will come to me at the right time."

Born in Oxnard, California, Cici has an interesting background of Mexican, Indian, Irish, and German. Her parents divorced when she was a child but remained in each other's lives. Her father, a World War II veteran, became a functioning alcoholic and died at age forty-eight of cirrhosis of the liver. Her mother remarried a widower with four children—an instant family merger with an active household. "It was so much fun," Cici laughed.

Cici became a bride when she and her husband, Rey, were both twenty years old, and they have had a strong marriage for forty-five years.

In 1977, when Cici was pregnant at age twenty-two, she developed a large ovarian cyst, and after exploratory surgery, she required blood transfusions. This was before blood banks tested for hepatitis C, and, unknown to anyone, the blood contained the virus. She carried her son to full term with no further complications, and she and Rey went on to have three more children.

When Cici complained of being tired and not feeling right in 1989, her doctors thought it was stress from her job. Two years later, she switched doctors and had liver tests. "And lo and behold," Cici said, "there it was—hepatitis C with cirrhosis of the liver and renal disease. My first reaction was that it was not true, that they had misdiagnosed me. They managed my disease with medication the best they could, but the more stress I was under at work, the more I got sick." Being promoted to director of human resources at several state-run facilities brought even more pressure.

She developed swollen veins in the esophagus, called varices, which burst causing her to cough up blood. Doctors did endoscopies each month and banded the varices to prevent bursting. After each procedure, she would take only one day off, even though it was extremely painful. Later, her boss tried to build a case against her, claiming Cici took off work too much, but the evidence proved otherwise.

Finally, the stress and her illness became too much, and in late 2009, Cici had a nervous breakdown. Driving home from work, she couldn't find her way, pulled over, and began crying hysterically. "It was a horrible feeling that came over me. Suddenly, I couldn't even remember how to drive a car. My husband and daughter came to get me and took me to the doctor. That's when I left work and never returned full-time," she said.

"I was still in denial of the severity of my health until the doctor told me the following year I had cancer of the liver. They did some chemo, but she said to me, 'Cici, you have a choice to live or die. I suggest you go to the Mayo Clinic because that's the best chance you have of living. If I list you here, you will not make it.'"

Rey was retired by then, and they went to Jacksonville in February 2011 for the Mayo testing but did not move there until a year later, when her cancer had grown to three tumors. They stayed at the Inn at Mayo, which was covered by their insurance company. She participated in the Second Chance Support Group, while they formed their own support group at the inn. "It felt like a family. We'd go out in the evenings, play games, bring home goodies, have pajama night. I had both kidney and liver disease, so I was on the transplant list for both. They never remove kidneys—they add a working one," she explained. "Many people don't know that."

Cici got the call from the procurement team on June 14, 2012. "As I was getting all my tests done before the late-night surgery, Father walked in and said that he felt the holy spirit in the room. On June 15, I had my kidney and first liver transplant," she said.

"Whenever you have a transplant with more than one organ, you must receive them from the same person," she went on. "Before every transplant, they thoroughly investigate the liver. But once they were doing my surgery, the antibodies were not matching, and complications were causing incompatibility. Essentially, they knew I would experience rejection of the liver so this became a temporary solution to my problem."

Cici was supposed to stay at Mayo after the transplant so she could be at the top of the list and quickly get another liver. But when the hospital called her insurance company, a doctor who took the call told Mayo to send her back to California, where she returned in August. "That was the worst call a doctor could have made," she said, "because once you leave the area, you do not remain in the same category on the waitlist anymore. You have to go through the whole process over again. So in October 2012, I went back to Mayo Clinic and waited twenty-two months for my next liver transplant!"

Instead of being angry that she had been sent back home prematurely, Cici grew emotional and said that God was taking care of her. "The second time around was the worst." She teared up. "But all that time I kept my faith. I knew I had to succeed and live for my family and myself. I was hospitalized, and they would take liters of fluid from my stomach. Water was seeping out of the pores of my legs and arms because it had nowhere else to go."

After a year of waiting in Jacksonville, Mayo wanted to send Cici back to California. However, her Kaiser doctor fought for her to stay, arguing that the reason she was waiting all this time was that she had been sent home too early.

"Rey always kept me going," Cici recalled. "People would come up to me and say, 'It's not fair. You've been here such a long time.' He recognized when I was falling into a downward spiral and lifted me up."

In November 2013, Cici finally got a call from Procurement saying, "We have a liver for you, but it is from a person who overdosed." HIPAA laws prevent recipients from knowing much information about the potential donor. The challenge, however, is that a recipient has to make a quick decision about accepting a high-risk liver.

Cici asked, "So how do I know if the person has HIV? If this person was out there wanting drugs or selling themselves to get drugs, that could make a difference."

"At this point in time, there is nothing there. We just know the death was from an overdose," the procurement representative said. "We wouldn't know if it had HIV until after transplant, and then it takes ten days to see if the liver would be working." With that limited information, they declined that liver and kept waiting.

Ten months later, in September 2014, Cici's body was beginning to shut down, and her MELD score rose from thirty-seven to forty-two. She was hospitalized for nine days receiving medications to stabilize her. No one told her what was going on—not even her husband—but she knew it was bad. She called her uncle, telling him it might be the last time she spoke to him.

"Sitting in a chair in the room was a man in a long, white gown with long hair, but I never saw his face," she remembered. "I was raised Catholic and have lots of faith. I thought I was imagining this. The image was only there for a second, but when I turned away and looked back, it was gone. I felt at peace. The next day, they drew my blood and told Rey that the blood count was getting better. I began to stabilize."

Three days later, Cici got a call saying the hospital had a liver for her, and she had her second transplant on September 7. "Afterwards, I did not bounce right back. Kaiser did not want me to return to California without ruling out all the possible problems, and my numbers were not leveling off, so I stayed in Jacksonville another five months," she explained. She was having rejection, which required several infusions and two liver biopsies. Finally, there was no more rejection, and she went home in February 2015.

But, back in California, the numbers started changing again. Kaiser and Mayo worked together, and Mayo suggested having a new biliary tube put in to drain toxins, which Kaiser did as an outpatient surgery. Three days later, Cici was in a fetal position with pain. "Apparently, when they inserted that wire, with such a narrow gap, the wire popped out, hitting something that gave me a hematoma on my left side," she said. "So now I had two bags outside of my body— one for the biliary tube and one for the hematoma." She spent thirty-two days in the hospital.

"Every three months, I had the biliary tube replaced while I was fully awake so I wouldn't have to stay in the hospital," she continued. When this was not rectifying the situation, doctors planned to send her back to Mayo. "They thought they could trim the liver, which would rejuvenate itself, and I would be fine. But after all the testing, it was determined that I needed another liver! That was the most devastating news I could have ever heard," she told me.

"I started the whole testing and waiting process all over again, but this time the liver had to be very specific. It had to have no antibodies and had to be from someone not over thirty years old. We knew it would be a long wait. After seventeen months, I started to feel the way I had before when I got real sick. At that stage, I told the doctors and everyone that I did not want to get to that point again because I did not think I could get through it. I don't know if you are aware, but every week at Mayo, the staff has a meeting. They pray for patients and put their names in a box. One of the nurses, Tiffany, told me they put my name in the box often," Cici recalled.

"In the eighteenth month, a woman called to say they had a liver and that they had all been praying for me to get one. I asked her if the person was thirty years old or younger. She said she could not answer that, but she could tell me that she herself was young. That was the clue I needed."

Doctors thought it would take eight to ten hours to do this transplant because of all the scar tissue. After only four hours of surgery, it was over. When she woke up, Rey asked her how she felt. Suddenly, Cici was overcome with emotion. "I feel alive!" she cried. "And that was the first time I said that. I felt my body totally awakened, not like the first or the second. I knew this was going to work. It was meant to be," she said, shaking as she remembered that moment. Doctors were amazed at how quickly she recuperated and how fast everything went back to normal.

"It was a miracle," she said, "because my journey has taught me to have more patience, to forgive, not argue, and to love life. My grandmother taught me to be kind throughout my life. When I saw people waiting and suffering because they wanted to go home, I faced them the same way my doctors faced me. You either want to live—and see your grandchildren grow up—or to die. You make that choice."

No matter how sick she was, she kept a smile on her face and tried to be there for others. She was there for so long that people would say, "Go to Cici. She'll help you."

"I can't thank the Mayo staff enough, They did so much. They cared so much. I still communicate with some of my nurses. My own doctor in L.A. fought for me. She pushed me because I didn't want to face what I had," Cici recalled. "The journey was hard, but it taught me so much. Look at every little detail. Slow life down, look and enjoy. Before, I was in the realm of working and constantly going and not really enjoying the moments. Now, you just don't take anything for granted. I take one day at a time and thank God for life. God only gives his journeys to the strongest warriors. I promised my kids I was going to beat this, and I did."

Cici concluded, "The true heroes in this story and every story are all the donors. Without them, none of this would be possible."

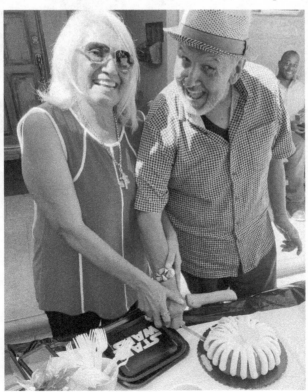

Cici and husband Rey

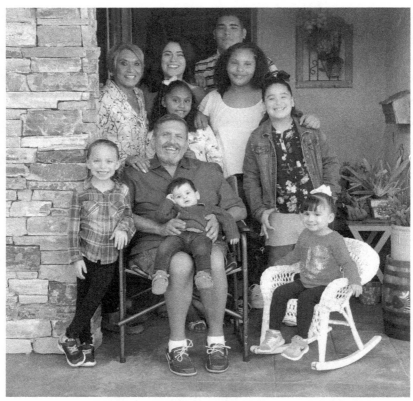

Cici, Rey and family

CHAPTER 28

Sarah: The Family Caregiver in Need of Caregiving

Our friend Jerry also suggested that I call Sarah, a young mother who suffered the same disease that Rob had.

Looking at Sarah's smiling, youthful face telling her story, it was hard to imagine that this wife and mother had needed a liver transplant when in her thirties. Her children had been ages eight and ten, and she had to put a family plan in place quickly so she could leave her home in California and travel to Jacksonville to have her life-saving surgery.

"My brother had offered to get tested to be my living donor," Sarah said. "But before we could even get started, my MELD score jumped from seventeen to twenty-one." Instead of risking two people's lives, doctors advised her to go to Florida, where she would have a better chance to receive a deceased donor liver.

"In October 2017, they wanted me to pack up and transfer to Mayo Clinic within two days. I panicked because I was a full-time mom with two kids in school, my husband was working, which also provided our benefits, and I didn't see how I could move across the country with hardly any notice," she said.

"The doctors made it clear that this was not a choice but my only option. They gave me one month to work out my schedule. So my parents lived in our home Monday through Thursday helping take care of the kids, my fellow 'mom friends' created a Friday pick-up/drop-off schedule at school,, and my husband took care of the children on weekends. My in-laws would relieve my parents when my ill father wasn't feeling well. Then, my mother's sister, Aunt Pam, agreed to come to Jacksonville and be my caregiver."

Sarah flew to Jacksonville on November 12. "Being away from my husband and children when I was their primary caregiver to suddenly needing a caregiver myself was devastating. The people at the Second Chance Support group became my surrogate family, which kept me going."

Growing up in Southern California, Sarah had rarely been sick, with "one heck of an immune system." She played sports and graduated in the top ten of her high school class.

During her freshman year at the University of California Riverside, she went to a Friday night party and met Jacob, who was in a neighboring dorm room. The next day he asked if she wanted to go to the dining room with him, but her meal plan was for weekdays only. He came back Sunday, but as it was still technically the weekend, he waited until Monday night to go to dinner with her. Her friends told her he was a keeper for trying so hard. They dated through college and married after graduation. Sarah became a fifth-grade teacher for three years until her son, Andrew, was born.

"I loved being in the classroom," she reflected. "My plan was to take a year off while he was a newborn, but then I got pregnant with my daughter, Allison. That pregnancy did not go as planned. I got extremely itchy to the point of tearing my skin off. The doctor thought it was cholangitis, a temporary flare-up of the liver, and would go away after I gave birth."

After delivery, the itching did not go away, and Sarah would wake up in a pool of sweat. She went to another specialist, who ordered further testing. At twenty-nine, with a toddler and newborn baby,

Sarah was diagnosed with primary sclerosing cholangitis (PSC). "That's when I started crying and didn't stop for years," she admitted.

"I did what every doctor tells you *not* to do—Google your disease, and it looked like a death sentence. It gave a seven- to ten-year downward spiral of liver failure. I thought I would not get to see my kids grow up or meet my grandkids and went into a depression with mood swings," she whispered.

In a brief interview, Jacob told me, "Yes, it was scary, but it also made us live differently. The fear of maybe not getting a transplant or not surviving made us go out of our way to do as much as we possibly could within our financial constraints."

"It did affect our intimacy, which is an important part of a relationship," Sarah admitted. "There was a lot of discussion, talking through our issues, and Jacob was incredibly understanding. He knew that between the side effects from my medication and feeling so tired all the time, it was hard for me to be in the mood. We are both grounded in Catholicism and believe you only marry once. Since divorce was not an option, and leaving him unhappy with all of his sacrifices was also not an option, we had to strive towards something that would work out for both of us."

Sarah discovered she also had ulcerative colitis. After taking too many sick days, she had to stop teaching full-time but could substitute teach. "I definitely did a lot of parenting from the couch," she admitted. "The kids got used to Jake being the more active parent. If they all wanted to take a hike, I would stay back and nap. To them, this was just part of their mom's life."

One of her bile ducts was completely blocked, so her doctors began stenting. "The problem was that once you introduce this invasive procedure, the stent has to be changed every three months. This went on for six years. As a result, I developed a buildup of scar tissue. This looked like cancer, so they sent me to the Mayo Clinic in Rochester where it was determined not to be cancer. They stopped stenting and let the disease take its course. I was taking a drug to slow down the progression, one to control the itching, sleeping aids, ulcerative colitis medicine, and a drug to control my moods," Sarah recalled.

"When I first got to the Mayo Clinic in Jacksonville, I was not in a good frame of mind, but I was not the only pouty person there," she admitted.

"Aunt Pam was attending the caregiver support group and encouraged me to go to the Second Chance Support Group, which was a turning point for me. I felt better listening to people who had struggles that were similar to mine. I didn't go to lunch with the group afterwards because I was bitter about having to be there and didn't want to engage too much, even though I connected with so many of them who were embracing and loving. They understood why I was so mad," Sarah said.

"It felt like I had an instant family when my immediate family was all gone. Lynn and Jerry were particularly so wonderful to me. Lynn gave me a rock in the shape of a liver that said 'courage' on it. Jerry and I were part of a knitting group where we knitted hats for children in Mexico."

Every time the phone rang, Sarah thought it was "the call." Her doctors kept telling her it's not "if," it's "when," and to be patient. Her husband and children came over for Christmas, and they celebrated it at the Mayo Inn. When the new year arrived in 2018, time slowed down, and the waiting was painful.

But then, on January 14 at 11:15 p.m., the phone rang when she least expected it. Two of her girlfriends with kids the same ages had happened to fly east to visit her, so she calls them her lucky charms.

"I hear you need a liver," the voice on the phone said.

"Oh, I do, I do, I do!" Sarah exploded.

"You sound pretty healthy. Are you sure you still need it?" he joked.

"Yes!" she shouted.

"Okay, we have one for you, but I want to give you a little

information so you can decide if you want it. It is a high-risk organ because the person had multiple sexual partners."

Sarah didn't even hesitate and said, "Well, who hasn't?" In her mind, everyone could be a high-risk liver.

Her friends helped her check into the hospital and even played hide-and-seek in the hospital room; when the nurse walked in, one friend was behind the IV stand and the other in the closet. The nurse patiently asked Sarah to lie down. "We wanted a girls' weekend," Sarah laughed. "We got an unexpected one. Everything fell into place, and I'm glad I had them there along with Aunt Pam, who I now have a lifelong bond with."

Due to a hold-up with the donor liver after she was at the hospital, the transplant was delayed until January 16.

"When I got the confirmation that the surgery was going through, I realized how lucky I was," Sarah acknowledged. "Going into this with religion helped me understand things in a different way. It has given me the sense to be patient and keep the faith even though it felt like my world was crumbling around me. I think God wanted me to be back with my husband and kids. Right before the surgery, I asked the doctor if he would take a picture of my liver, and he did! It looked like a black, charred bun cake.

"I immediately felt so much better post-transplant. Suddenly, my organs were working properly, but I must say the medication can mess with your head. Sometimes it is physical and other times mental. You have to overcome these obstacles."

Today, she goes whitewater rafting and zip-lining with her family. She can participate and be the active mom her kids deserve.

"I equate my transplant to giving birth to a child, where you forget all the pain and relish this new life. We are in full swing of family activities and I'm not dwelling on the past. Thankfully, we have moved forward. I didn't realize how sick I was until after transplant. I feel like my kids got the mom they should have had to begin with," she said. "In terms of COVID, I take precautions, but I'm so happy about living that I am not going to live in fear. I'm having one hell of a parade and not letting anything rain on it!"

Sarah continues to praise her husband. "Jacob is probably one of the most patient and understanding people you will ever meet. I don't feel it was by chance that this guy was put into my life. I feel like he was thrown to me by God. I don't know if our marriage would have thrived the way it did with anyone else. You have to stay on the rollercoaster ride because the good parts are worth staying for."

She feels strongly that she has to continue the legacy of her donor, whoever he or she is. She writes a yearly letter to her donor family but fears she might be in the seventy-five percent of recipients who do not hear back.

"Many times the donor's family cannot accept someone's else's happiness over the pain of their loss. I have to remember how I might feel if my child died and another person was benefiting from my loss. I completely understand both sides. It would be such a waste to take this liver and mope around with it. Yes, I am sad for the donor who lost his life, but I am so happy to be alive because of their gift."

Feeling she has a responsibility to honor this person's life, she joined the Donate Life Ambassador program in California. She speaks to new-hire nurses in hospitals on the value of talking with families about organ donation. And because she loves teaching, she talks to high school students who are getting their driver's licenses and explains how important it is to check that organ donor box.

"The people I have met through the Donate Life organization have become my new support group," Sarah concluded. "Whether they are a donor family, a recipient, or a living donor, we are all for the common good of promoting organ donation. Right now, I am lucky that I get to serve the world in the way that I want to. My job is to honor myself and my donor by being loving and caring, living my life to the fullest while being grateful and joyful."

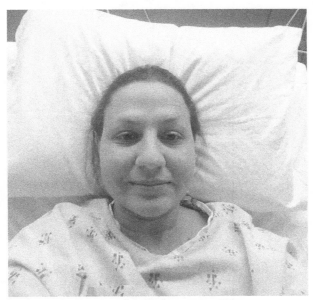

Sarah in hospital pre-transplant

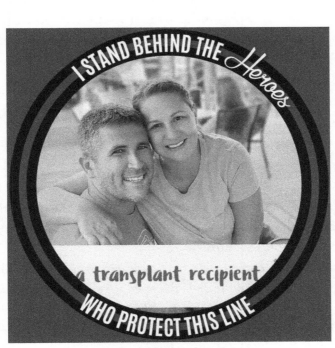

Sarah and husband Jacob

CHAPTER 29

Changes on the Homefront

September 2020, St. Augustine and Nyack

Since launching the petition to UNOS, there had been some changes in our lives. The biggest one was that, after begging us all summer, River flew home to Nyack. We knew that he would do better in school if he was in his own environment. So he returned August 27, stayed first with Rob's brother, John Paul, and then at our neighbor Anna's house until our summer renters left. Finally, River slept in his own bed while our friends Mostafa and Lobna stayed at our home with their seven-year-old daughter, Amira, and Salem, River's closest friend. Lobna, who grew up in Egypt, made traditional meals, and River ate like a king.

It is not easy to find a family willing to take in your child or live in your home to oversee them indefinitely. But luckily, our friends and neighbors were following our story and wanted to help in any way they could. When you ask for what you need, you might be surprised at people's generosity.

Meanwhile, I learned that my bedridden, eighty-year-old father had stopped eating, and the day I dropped River off at the Jacksonville airport, I drove six hours to Atlanta with Skye to spend what I thought were the last moments of my dad's life with him. Even though Dad was sleeping most of the time and could not speak or move much, I told him all about Rob. Somehow, he rallied, maybe to know what would happen, or maybe just to have a little more time.

I had planned to stay a week in Atlanta and be back for Rob's upcoming endoscopy, but seeing Dad in such a state, I was torn whether to leave him or not. It was my father's sister, my beloved Aunt Dale, who gave me important advice. Married to Dr. Jerry Goldsmith, a retired orthopedic surgeon, she had also lived inside the world of medicine and been my uncle's caregiver when he overcame pancreatic cancer.

"Your father is in good hands," she told me. "You need to go back to Florida and be with your husband. He needs you." She was right.

Rob had his endoscopy September 4 while I waited in the hospital. Doctors inserted a tube down his throat and put small rubber bands around the varicose veins inside his esophagus, cutting off the blood supply to keep them from bursting; if they did, he could bleed to death.

After Rob came out from the anesthesia, the nurse told me that he had such excruciating pain in his chest that they wanted to admit him overnight for pain management. I did not expect this. She let me go back and see him, and he was miserable. The next day, when I picked him up, he needed strong pain meds and could barely eat anything. We were told that he'd have to have this procedure again in six weeks. The thought of that made Rob so upset. The pain was only beginning.

At this point, the dark circles under Rob's eyes combined with his jaundice and fatigue made him look deathly ill. I could barely remember him any other way.

The first time I heard Luigi's voice describe his circumstances on the virtual support group, I wanted to hear his story. Despite what he was facing, he had such a positive outlook. Rob, on the other hand, was losing hope so I wanted them to connect.

Another interesting transplant patient was Kathy, one of the first people Rob met at the in-person support group. She was on the liver transplant wait list too, but unlike Rob, she did not have to wait that long for transplant.

Meet Luigi and Kathy in the next chapters.

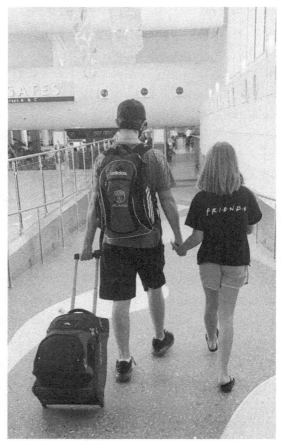

River and Skye walking hand and hand at airport

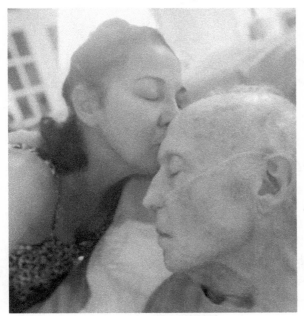

Lezlee kissing her father

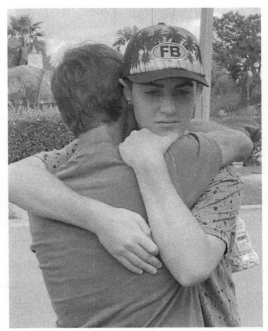

Saying goodbye to Dad

CHAPTER 30

Luigi: The 'Luckiest Man on Earth'

"Time is a priceless commodity," said Luigi, also called Luis, with his slight Mexican accent as he handed Rob a custom watch from one liver transplant patient to another. "Time is something we both appreciate and need more of." Luigi describes himself as "the luckiest man on earth." After hearing his story, I understood why.

Raised in an affluent home in the outskirts of Mexico City, Luigi is the free-spirited eldest of four. He is tall, with a commanding voice and a positive outlook on life. His father founded a manufacturing company that supported at least sixty local families working there. "I was privileged without being spoiled," Luigi said.

"My dad wanted me to work in the factory starting at the bottom like everyone else, study, and do things his way, but I am not good at taking orders," he admitted. "We butted heads when I was a teenager, and in anger, he told one of the maids to pack my things, put them in my car, and told me, 'The day you become a man of good, you are welcome in this house.' So, I left home when I was seventeen and never returned." For a while, he was homeless, sleeping under a bridge, on the streets, and picking up food from trash containers.

Luigi survived by doing all kinds of work in the service industry, later traveling back and forth from Mexico to Los Angeles catering events. Mostly, he worked for himself and slowly built up a sales career. "I was young, having fun, and learned how to take care of myself," he explained. "It's called the University of Life." Eventually, he and his father began communicating again, and their relationship healed.

In 1997, Luigi was working as a "gentle organizer" (GO) at the Club Med resort in Cancun. One day, he spotted a beautiful young woman who was there on vacation. Daniella had grown up in Lebanon but now lived in London. A kindergarten teacher, she had only two days left before returning home. "When I saw Daniella, I knew that this was a train I needed to get on," Luigi said with a grin.

"I noticed Luigi, but he was not my type. He had long, curly hair and was very serious, never smiled," Daniella recounted. "But something about him attracted me."

After she returned to London, Luigi sent her flowers with a note, "This Mexican GO misses you."

"I did the craziest thing of my life," Daniella admitted. "Just two months later, in July, I went all the way across the world by myself to see him again."

After some ups-and-downs and misunderstandings, Luigi asked her to come to Mexico City to meet his parents. He quit his job, and they flew out the next morning.

Daniella felt a cultural kinship with Luigi's family because of her Mediterranean and German background. "Being with his family reminded me of our way of living," she said. She went home after ten days, and Luigi traveled to London the following month. "He proposed in the most romantic way," Daniella joked. "While I was on the white commode throne!"

"It just highlighted the craziness of our story," Luigi laughed. They were married in London in October, and Daniella got pregnant on her wedding night. Suddenly, their travel and party plans changed.

"Who cares about planning?" Luigi recounted. "Life is one day at a time."

They moved to Mexico and, after a lovely church wedding in the town of Taxco, they began their life together in Cuernavaca.

On July 6, 1998, their daughter Vanessa was born. That was the last day Luigi's father left the house; he had battled for several years with both colon and liver cancer. He went to the hospital to see his granddaughter, saying, "Some new lives arrive, and some old lives are ready to go."

Luigi's father had made some poor decisions in his last year, when he did not have the strength to battle certain family members who took control of his company. What Luigi later realized was that one potential effect of end-stage liver disease is that patients often do not make clear decisions because their liver is not processing toxins, which clouds their judgment.

In a twist of fate, at the end of 1998 soon after his father died, Luigi began to feel tired with pain on the upper right side of his liver. A hepatologist in Mexico diagnosed him with hepatitis B and C, explaining that eventually he would need a transplant. He immediately went to the Mayo Clinic in Jacksonville, where Dr. Spivey, who had performed his father's liver recession two years earlier, was now director of the liver transplant team. At the time, Luigi had excellent private health insurance, which Mayo Clinic accepted.

"Your liver does not look that bad," Dr. Spivey told him. "Down the line, you might need a transplant, but for now, no drinking alcohol, and we should just keep an eye on it every six months."

Given the potential for Luigi's health deterioration, Daniella was worried about having more children, but in 2001, they had a second daughter, Valerie. The family was living in Mexico, traveling frequently.

At a regular Mayo Clinic checkup in 2005, Luigi's hepatologist, Dr. Raj, brought concerning news. "Your liver now has cirrhosis with a lesion. We would like you to relocate to Jacksonville and be on the active transplant list."

Luigi sold almost everything the family had, and they moved. "We had a little bit of savings, and I began selling things on eBay," he said. "We had a tourist visa. Our daughters and Daniella are German citizens through Daniella's father, so every ninety days, they were required to leave the United States."

Flying to Mexico every three months became expensive, so Luigi created his own company that designed watches. He had to prove that he had a background in jewelry through his grandmother, who had been a well-known silversmith, even designing a necklace for Eleanor Roosevelt. This business enabled them to obtain a NAFTA visa and remain in the U.S legally.

As Luigi was prone to tuberculosis, doctors began treating him with isoniazid, an antibiotic. Within weeks, he developed isoniazid liver failure, and his body became yellow with jaundice. The surgeon was pushing for an immediate transplant with a possible "second-grade liver," but Dr. Raj wanted to see if Luigi's liver would correct itself on its own. After stopping this medicine, his liver naturally recovered, and they took him off the transplant waitlist.

"At that point, I was very sick and needed help doing basic things," Luigi remembered. "But I said to Daniella, before I die, let's make love one more time. I've never planned anything in my whole life, and unexpectedly, Daniella became pregnant again." They went to see a doctor to assess the risks of complications for the baby based on Luigi's medications. He was having plasma transfusions and taking a drug called interferon with terrible side effects. Thankfully, the doctor said, "God sends miracles at the strangest times in the strangest ways. Your baby is fine."

Luigi told Dr. Raj that he was quitting all the aggressive drugs he was taking to control the hepatitis because he simply wanted to enjoy being an active father. "This is not something you want to mess around with," Dr. Raj said. But Luigi wanted to make the most of his life. His son, Luigi Jr., was born December 8, 2006, on the birthday of Luigi's father.

Several years went by. The family moved to a small house near Houston, Texas, and stopped travel, except for going to Mayo Clinic for yearly checkups. "Even though I knew it would be a huge financial cost, I decided not to work much because I wanted to be at every school event and every milestone in our children's lives," Luigi said.

In 2013, Daniella began working in real estate, and with mounting legal fees to extend and reapply for their visas, they were considering moving to Germany or Mexico. Then something happened that changed their fate.

"Instead of planning ahead, I ended up *planting* ahead," Luigi said, laughing. "Many years ago, way before I met Daniella, I had a brief affair with a woman in Los Angeles. Facebook had just become popular, and I got a message from this woman telling me that her twenty-year-old son, named Luis Carlos, was hanging out with the wrong crowd and had just been shot—and that he was my son! After much thought, I decided to contact him. While we could not go back and change the past, I invited him to meet and build a fresh relationship so we could be part of each other's lives now. This is one of the best decisions I have made. Luis Carlos, my eldest son, has a great heart and is a good kid."

Luigi learned that his name was on the birth certificate, and because his son had been a minor at the time he and Daniella married, she was legally considered his stepmother. Therefore, both Luigi and Daniella could become legal residents of the United States; soon they will be able to apply for U.S. citizenship.

Luigi's health remained stable until early 2020, when he was rushed to the ER with terrible pain. Daniella had a new job in the relocation industry with health insurance benefits, so she was able to add Luigi. The doctor came in and, in front of their children, told them that Luigi not only had a kidney stone, he also had liver cancer with three lesions. Luigi turned around to see Daniella and his daughters crying but assured them that he would be okay.

In April 2020, Luigi rekindled his relationship with Mayo Clinic and began going back and forth from Houston to Jacksonville for treatments. In May, he had a minimally invasive procedure targeting two of his tumors. In June, before having an ablation to destroy abnormal tissue, Luigi tested positive for COVID-19. The doctor was kind enough to go ahead and do the procedure by putting him in a special room before the anesthesia.

The three lesions were gone by the end of June. Following protocol set by UNOS, Luigi had to wait six months after treatment of cancerous tumors to obtain exception points allowing him to be actively listed for liver transplant.

On December 22, 2020, his exception points kicked in, raising his MELD score from seven to twenty-two, an acceptable number for transplant. The entire family flew to Jacksonville, including Daniella's mother, her brother, and sister-in-law, and rented a home near the Mayo Clinic. Miraculously, Luigi was called for transplant the very next day.

In an interview with him shortly before his transplant, he told me, "I am the luckiest man on earth. My father's liver surgery at Mayo Clinic in Rochester led me to come to Mayo Clinic in Jacksonville. Meeting Daniella was winning the lottery. We've been married twenty-three years and have a wonderful family. I've always been a positive person, believing that everything happens for a reason. I'm not worried because the universe has a plan that things happen at the right place at the right time."

On Christmas morning, Luigi received his liver transplant. Everything went well, and he was released from the hospital on schedule. "I was put on steroids right after surgery," he explained, "and I felt like hunting lions in the forest. I was eating well, walking around, and feeling great."

At a follow-up visit, Luigi asked to see the pathology report of his old liver. Afterwards, they discovered something unbelievable. Hidden from all the previous scans taken was a fourth lesion on the back of his liver. "Once again, I am the luckiest man on earth because had this tumor been detected, I would not have been a candidate for transplant," Luigi explained. Having more than three tumors disqualifies a patient today.

Nothing seemed out of the ordinary. Until it wasn't...

A month after his surgery, Luigi began to have excruciating pain. After many tests, he was admitted to the hospital with an elevated temperature, and doctors detected poor blood flow going to his liver. They tried procedures including an angiogram to unblock the vein. Then, Dr. Nguyen, who performed Luigi's liver transplant, had to deliver unfortunate news. "He explained that I had something called hepatic artery stenosis, which means when they closed, somehow one of the arteries was pinched. The only way to fix it was to go back in, and it would be even more complicated than a liver transplant."

This surgery took longer than the transplant had. "I had no choice but to have this, but I was not prepared for the toll it would take on my body," Luigi admitted. "The constant pain was unbelievable, and I spent many nights crying. The macho was certainly taken away from this Mexican. At first, I was angry. I was a few days from going home, feeling great, and then everything started going wrong. Why was this happening to me? Financially, it was a burden. I felt so guilty because my whole family team was stuck here because of me. For the first time since my illness, I had no input in my care. I have always been a patient who wants to discuss options, but I was too weak."

After leaving the hospital, he had to return a short time later with severe pain. A tiny hole between the donor's bile duct and his own had caused a staph infection. "Bile is so acidic and aggressive that my body protected itself with water, and I could feel my lungs filling up," he said. "It was a struggle to breathe." Doctors put him on round-the-clock antibiotics with a drain to prevent sepsis. When he was released again, he still had IVs in him.

"We had to stay near the Mayo Clinic until the bile drain had healed," Daniella chimed in during our video interview. "Administering Luigi's two IVs by myself was a nightmare. I set alarms for everything. One of them was administered every twelve hours and took two hours to empty. The other one was every six hours and lasted an hour. Neither one of could sleep much at all."

"I was just waiting for Daniella to put on that kinky nurse outfit," Luigi joked.

"That was not going to happen," she responded, smiling.

On March 11, Luigi had another angiogram done to fix the stenosis; he also had an aneurism of the liver. Doctors placed a stent in the donor vein because it was collapsing; this procedure made him feel much better. "I was one hundred percent dependent on Daniella," Luigi confessed. "My concern was that she needed to recharge her battery. The caregivers have such a special role and need their own support group. I look forward to my Tuesday virtual support group meetings."

Finally, Luigi's body began to heal, and he was able to go home. While transplant patients usually reach out to their donor families six months post-transplant, Luigi actually received a letter from his donor's family, and they have been corresponding.

"The universe aligns things," Luigi concluded. "If you look back on all the small things that occurred, it was all meant to happen. I am grateful to be among the very few people in this world who have been given a second chance through transplant."

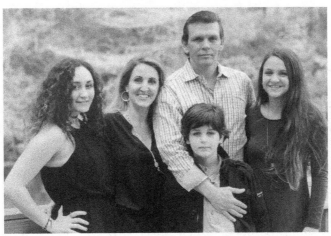

Luigi, Daniella and family

CHAPTER 31

Kathy: How Could Someone Be So Sick, Yet Asymptomatic?

"When I was first diagnosed with non-alcoholic cirrhosis in 2014, I joined a few online support groups," Kathy confessed, "but I had to quit them because I felt horribly guilty for the terrible things people were going through that I was not experiencing. Even though I had the same disease, I had virtually no symptoms except my stomach felt like I had acid reflux, which was what led me to seek a doctor. I couldn't relate to what doctors were telling me was actually happening inside my body. That's why it is so important to go to a doctor to get regular checkups or to get an answer to even a small problem."

Kathy had arrived at the Mayo Clinic in October 2019, about the same time as Rob, and they met each other through the Second Chance Support Group meetings. They had the same O blood type. Kathy was lucky and received her liver transplant a few weeks after she arrived, but her MELD score was higher than Rob's.

Kathy grew up in California in the 1950s. Her father, a World War II veteran, owned a barber shop, and her mother was a beautician whose clients came to the family's home. Later, they opened a jewelry store in Santa Barbara, which succeeded for many years. After high school, Kathy became a bookkeeper, office manager, then a comptroller for a petroleum company, working there sixteen years.

She met her first husband in 1968 and got married a year later. They had a son, Sean, and were married for twenty-two years. "You know how they say that life begins at forty," Kathy joked. "Well, for me, I had a hysterectomy, divorce, carpal tunnel on both wrists, and a biopsy of my breast, so my health struggles began at forty."

Two years after her divorce, she met Bill, and they dated for five years before marrying in 1998. Bill had six children, so it became an instant blended large family.

Other than her weight, Kathy had no major health problems for many years. She was never a big drinker. "I realized early on that if I drank, I'd miss out on all the fun," she laughed, "because the alcohol just made me sleepy."

Bill was a general contractor, and the couple owned their own business. They had small business health insurance with Kaiser, which was affiliated with Mayo Clinic. From commercial buildings, they changed to building houses in 2003, doing quite well until the housing market crashed. After that, Bill got a job with Home Depot, and Kathy went back to work. When Bill had been with Home Depot a year, he was able to buy the company's stock at a discounted price. The company also paid for Bill's health insurance and part of Kathy's. Together, they recovered, saved money, and moved on.

Then, out of nowhere, Kathy began to have some minor stomach-related issues. She was treated for acid reflux, and doctors first thought she had a hiatal hernia, an ulcer, or gastroesophageal reflux disease. "Around 2010, first thing in the morning, I would have a dry heave, and then it was over with," she remembered. "It didn't happen a whole lot, but I thought it was odd. Then it started happening more regularly. One day when I was going to work, I had to stop the car because I started vomiting."

Her doctor ordered an ultrasound in 2014 and found she had cirrhosis of the liver. When she'd had lab work done in the past, nothing showed up. Kathy had no idea how she went from having acid reflux and heartburn to cirrhosis of the liver!

Doctors wanted to do an esophagogastroduodenoscopy (EGD) to examine the esophagus, stomach, and first portion of the small intestine, using an endoscope with a camera on a flexible tube inserted in the mouth.

"I have a phobia of choking," Kathy admitted. "The first time I went in to have it done, it freaked me out." She had esophageal varices, enlarged veins on the lining of the esophagus, caused by cirrhosis. The doctor explained that they could start bleeding, unknown to her, or she could begin coughing up blood, and it would be too late—she could bleed out in front of her family. "I knew I didn't want that, so I faced my fear and had the EGD," she said.

For the procedure, Kathy had to lie on her side, with a guard placed in her mouth to keep it open, and then was put in a twilight sleep because she had to follow directions and swallow the camera. When the medical team saw varices, another instrument was put down with small rubber bands to band the varices so they would disappear. She had thirty-two EGDs in four years.

"When they banded the varices the first time," Kathy recalled, "I truly thought I was going to choke to death. Afterwards, the pain right between my breasts hurt incredibly bad. No one prepared me for that. It was hard to eat and drink from the irritation of this foreign object in my esophagus." Finally, a year before her transplant, she had no more varices.

In general, Kathy felt fine and still couldn't believe something terrible was wrong with her. She was working and enjoying her family. For two years, she had regular MRIs done, and in 2016, her doctor called to say there was a small lesion on her liver. "When they told me I had a tumor, it sent me into a tailspin. Again, I had no symptoms," Kathy said. She was sent to the cancer tumor board in Los Angeles and made the three- to four-hour trip there every few months to have her condition monitored.

Ironically, she had to wait until the cancer grew before they could do anything about it. Without the cirrhosis, doctors could have done a biopsy or even removed the lesion because the liver regenerates itself. Because she had cirrhosis that had damaged her liver so badly, there was no way they could take the cancer out.

In January 2019, after another MRI, doctors saw that her cancer had indeed grown. "When the doctor called, he asked me if I wanted a liver transplant. I asked if there was another option, and he said, 'Not really.' I began the transplant evaluation at Los Angeles Kaiser, and they approved me even though they don't do transplants. They talked about other associated hospitals in California, but the transplant waitlist time there could be three to five years and I might not have lived that long. They suggested Mayo Clinic in Florida. I said, 'Of course.' I didn't want to be that far away from my family, especially not knowing how long it could be, but I knew Mayo was an outstanding medical facility, and I would do anything for more time with my family."

She and her husband came to Jacksonville on April 14. "We were there for two weeks, and I had so many tests, some of the same and some new and very different," she said.

"Everyone we dealt with made me feel that they absolutely had my best health in mind. The grounds at Mayo are like a wonderful resort. There is an island between the medical buildings that I called 'Sanctuary Island' because it was peaceful and comforting. I spent many hours there. At the end of all the testing and appointments, I was approved for a transplant. Because of my weight, they wanted me to do a bariatric sleeve surgery to cut away eighty percent of my stomach at the same time as the transplant. My weight has been a challenge most of my life, but I wanted to live, so I was open to all options."

When she returned to California at the end of April, she had six months before heading back to Mayo and needed to attend twelve weeks of bariatric classes, continue labs and procedures, but, most importantly, deal with her cancer. In June, she had her first treatment by a radiologist who injected chemotherapy directly into the tumor via the femoral artery.

"After this procedure, we found out that I had three tumors. In July, I had another MRI, and the tumors had not shrunk enough, so they scheduled another treatment. On my seventieth birthday in July, Sean and his wife, Lindy, and my cousin, Linda, threw me a huge surprise party! So many family and friends came, and it was wonderful with so much love." Kathy beamed at the memory.

"By August, after another treatment, they found two more tumors, so I had a total of five," she recounted. She had to lie flat on her back for four hours after the chemotherapy procedure. After lying there about forty-five minutes, she went into full body tremors. "I had no idea what was happening and thought I was going to die. The doctor gave me something to ease the tremors. It worked, but this happened two more times," she said.

"I knew the healthier I would be going into my surgery, the better my results. I started fitness training two or three times a week and discovered I enjoyed it. The bariatric classes were also teaching me a healthier way to eat. After six months, I lost fifty pounds on my own and was officially placed on the Mayo Clinic transplant list, and I did not need bariatric surgery!" Kathy declared proudly.

When she went back to the Mayo Clinic, she had a MELD score of seventeen, and exception points for the cancer brought it up to twenty-five. Rob was listed with a MELD score of nineteen.

"The first support meeting I went to," Kathy said, "I met Captain Rob. We were the only pre-transplant patients. Then there was another woman also waiting on a liver, but she was much sicker than I was and in the hospital for two weeks before her transplant."

Her insurance coverage included housing, and Kathy was staying on campus at the Marriott. "Early Saturday morning on November 9, only two weeks after my arrival, I walked over to the island. I needed to have a talk with God. I believe He has a plan for each of us. I was missing my family horribly."

Kathy got her procurement call that same day at 3 p.m. "We think we have a liver for you," the transplant coordinator told her, "And we will give you a call back between 5 and 7 p.m., so please have your bag packed." Soon, the second call came, and she went to the ER to get admitted.

"It was so incredible. I felt so good about everything and had a real calmness about myself. Dr. Croome was my surgeon, and I thought he was absolutely adorable. I remember going into the operating room at 11 p.m. and hearing him say that the liver had arrived, and it was a go. They put the mask on my face, and I counted backwards from ten; at nine, I was out. The next thing I knew, on November 10, they were waking me up telling me it was over. I honestly hardly had any pain afterwards," Kathy recalled.

"My only symptoms from all the medicine I'm taking now are that my body feels like it is on a low vibrate, and I've had some full tremors as well. There are places on my body that are totally numb, and since I have to give myself insulin shots as a diabetic, it's the greatest thing because I don't feel anything," she laughed.

Together, she and Bill have sixteen grandchildren, one great-grandchild, and a great-grandchild on the way. Unfortunately, the coronavirus changed life. "My kids have been scared they are going to infect me." Kathy's voice broke. "And that really bothers me. I was expecting to wear a mask and be careful, but to come back to all of this is unreal. My eldest grandchildren understand, but my youngest doesn't know why she can't come up on my lap and hug me. It adds another dimension to the return."

She has found the support group Zoom meetings very helpful. "The doctors and nurses are wonderful, but when you go to a support group, the pre- and post-transplant patients are talking because they have been there, done that. We have lived through this incredible experience," Kathy said.

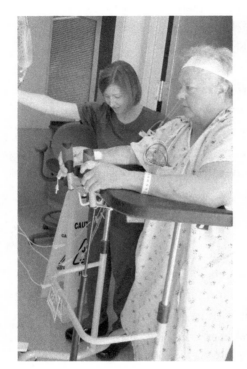 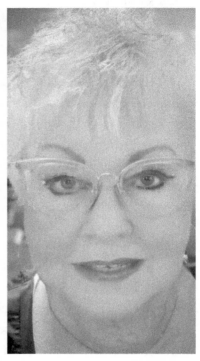

Kathy in the hospital, November 2019, and now at home in California

CHAPTER 32

Rob Finally Gets His Liver Transplant!

September 2020, St. Augustine

September 9 was the first day of school. In the morning, Anna, my friend and neighbor in Nyack, sent me a picture of River sitting at her living room table next to her son, Dylan, with their computers and headphones beginning their sophomore year. Because of COVID, the schools were opening virtually for the first three weeks.

Skye, now attending Nyack Public Middle School as a sixth grader through remote learning, was able to participate from her room in St. Augustine. I spent most of the day resting on Skye's bed while she was at her desk doing Zoom classes with her teachers.

We spoke to Rob's liver coordinator in the morning, and I told her how defeated we were feeling. We were supposed to go to Mayo the next day and see another hepatologist about the results of his recent endoscopy. Rob was hungry so I made him a sandwich. Suddenly, I heard a big *boom*. I ran into the other room, and he said he had passed out from pain in his chest resulting from the procedure he had undergone a few days before. He moved to the sofa, and I put a cold compress on his head.

That evening, I was watching an old episode of the medical drama *Grey's Anatomy* in Skye's room on my computer. Ironically, the show we were watching happened to feature a patient needing a liver transplant.

At 11:30, Rob came into the room. A woman from Procurement had just called, saying there were two livers, and one of the intended recipients might not match the size of the organ. It took a minute for me to process, but I didn't get that excited. We had been through this before.

Then, shortly after midnight, I got into bed with Rob, and the phone rang again. Rob picked it up and put it on speaker.

"Hi, Rob. This is Inga from Procurement. The liver is going to you. This is a good liver. There are no high risks. How quickly can you get to the hospital?"

At 12:15 a.m., Rob and I got in the car, with the sky flashing lightning bolts and the rain pouring down. We reached the ER at 12:58 a.m., checked in, and followed a nurse up to room 317. Rob went through the same prep as he had done before except this time, the anesthesiologist came in to talk to us, and then we met with the surgeon, Dr. Shennen Mao.

A few hours passed, and nurses came in with a wheelchair to take him to the operating room.

Finally, it was all coming together.

"How do you feel, Rob?" I asked him.

"I feel ready."

"Don't forget to take a picture of my liver," Rob reminded one of the nurses. A nurse said they would call me on the hospital phone to give updates.

As they were wheeling Rob off, I felt so keyed up that I burst into the song I had written and performed at an event for the American Liver Foundation.

Be a giver of your liver when it's time to go
And you can help lots of people that you may not know
Don't be afraid to give
So someone else can live
Be a giver of your liver when it's time to go

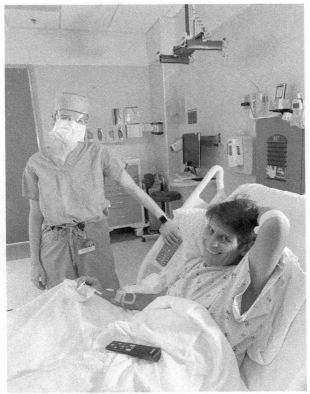

First meeting with Dr. Mao

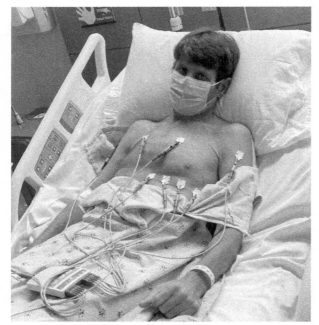

Testing just before surgery

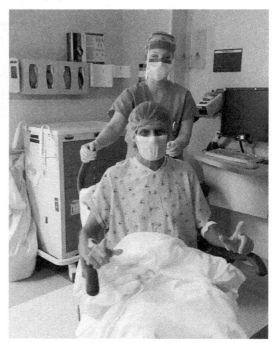

Wheeled off to surgery

CHAPTER 33

My Notes During the Transplant: Day One

5:15 a.m. — I am lying down on hospital guest sofa in the room waiting to hear some news. I have spoken to no one in my family yet. Suddenly the phone rings, and I jump up to answer it. "Mrs. Bellanich, this is the nurse in the OR. I just want to let you know that the doctor has made the first incision, and your husband is doing very well so far." That's all I need to hear.

5:30 a.m. — I figure it's time to let some family know what is going on, so I send a text to Rob's brothers and sisters-in-law telling them that Rob just began his transplant surgery! It's still early so no one responds.

7:30 a.m. — The phone rings, and the nurse tells me that they have removed Rob's liver ... OMG. I have an image of him lying on the bed with tubes and machines keeping him alive while they scoop out his diseased liver and put it ... where? in a dish? I'm not sure. I can't take it anymore. I need to call someone, so I call my brother Scott.

"It's a little early for you, isn't it?" he answers.

"Well, I just wanted to let you know that we are at the Mayo Clinic and Rob is halfway through his liver transplant surgery."

"What? Are you kidding me?" Scott shouts. "Why didn't you call me earlier?"

"I wanted to make sure it was a go and didn't want you to be awake the whole night like me."

"Who is with Skye?"

"No one. She is still asleep."

"Well, I am going to grab a few things and drive to you," he insists. "It will take me about five or six hours from Atlanta." God, I love my brother! When push comes to shove, he drops everything without having to be asked.

9 a.m. — Another call comes in. "Hi, I just wanted to let you know that the new liver is in Rob, and the doctor has connected the arteries. She is going to do a procedure to re-route the donor's bile duct, which will take another hour. We should close at 11 o'clock, and then he will be in the recovery room until about noon."

"Then he comes back to this room?" I ask.

"Yes."

Wow! They aren't even taking him to the ICU. So, I wait. The texts come in from concerned family and friends. Soon, they come in to get Rob's hospital bed to transfer him. I can't wait to see him.

11:15 a.m. — I recognize the woman coming into the room with her mask. It's Dr. Mao! "He did great," she says. "Everything went exactly as we expected it to. We took out the old liver. It was definitely sick, very swollen and scarred. It looked like a liver that had PSC because they are often blobby and swollen, especially the right lobe. Then we put the new liver in its place. It's a nice liver, and we made all those connections we talked about. His bile duct did not look quite right so it was safest to do the *Roux-en-Y*, where we took out the bile duct he was born with and made another connection from his intestine and the donor liver to create a new duct to drain bile."

She tells me that an ultrasound will be done to see if there is anything concerning. "It looked good when we finished," she said, "so I don't think there will be any troubles, but we always check that as a routine."

I thank her from our entire family.

About 12:15 p.m. — The door opens, and Rob is wheeled in with tubes coming from his nose, the side of his neck, and chest .... He is flat on his back with his eyes mostly closed, but he suddenly looks better to me. I stare down at him so he can see my face.

"I love you, Lez," he mumbles. "Thank you for sticking by me."

Wow. Those few words fill my heart. I am not even sure he will remember saying that to me, but I needed to hear it.

"The pain," he mumbles, "the pain." Rob is holding a white instrument with a green circle in his hand. The nurse tells him to press it when he needs pain medicine. It will allow the appropriate amount to pass through his IV.

Slowly, nurses begin working on him as I sit there watching in awe. About an hour later, technicians come in with an ultrasound machine to check the liver ... Rob's mouth is so dry, and I get a swab with water to brush it across his lips, and he sucks on it. The room feels hot and he is sweating, so I get a wet washcloth and put it over his forehead. It hurts watching him in pain trying to regain consciousness. He wants me to take pictures so he can see for himself later. He also knows that documenting this is important.

Finally, Rob seems more awake. His color looks better than before. The new liver is processing the toxins, and his yellow eyes become lighter and whiter. He looks at me with a more relaxed look, even gives me a slight smile. This sight is truly unbelievable!

Scott decides to drive directly to St. Augustine to cook and take care of Skye.

Having been awake for about thirty-two hours, I figure out how to open the sofa bed and begin writing my first Facebook post with pictures to document the ordeal. So many people have been following our story, and we need to communicate how important this subject is.

While some folks may have cringed at the details, my mind is clear. I know that if people truly understand that without donors, none of this would be possible, all of this will be worth it.

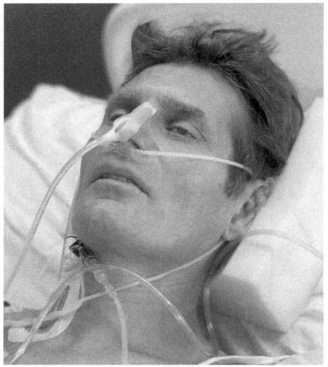

First look after transplant surgery

CHAPTER 34

Notes from the First Week

September 11, Day 2 after Captain Rob's Miraculous Liver Transplant

Warning: Some of the images and descriptions that follow could either be fascinating or gory depending on your perspective. Once you keep reading, there's no turning back! Rob wanted me to record everything because we are now educators and advocates through this incredible process.

Think of science class when they made you dissect a frog. There is a lot to learn when it comes to anatomy ...

Today there were so many happenings and incredible realizations.

We were as prepared as we could be going into this transplant because of the friendships we have made through the Second Chance Support Group. But nothing truly prepares you until you go through it. And every day is something new.

This is an intense subject that we should not fear but rather celebrate. It's like mad science on steroids. Here are notes from the experience:

- 5:30 a.m.: Rob calls out to me while I am asleep on the pullout bed because the nurses want him to sit and then stand up for the first time, which he does. Then, a few hours later, with the assistance of occupational and physical therapists, he walks around the whole floor with a rolling walker! Nurses and doctors say he is doing incredibly well.

- 9 a.m.: The color in Rob's face has returned along with the whites of his eyes. The new liver is working beautifully.

- Even though Rob is in pain from being cut (mostly into his stomach muscles) and in need of rest, it is a different kind of tired from what he had been experiencing before. With PSC, for years and years, he felt like he was always carrying a heavier and heavier anchor around him. "Now the anchor line has been cut, and I feel free!" he just said.

- During Rob's surgery, we learned, there were two liver transplants going on at once, and the anesthesiologist had to oversee both at the same time, going back and forth between the two operating rooms.

- The main reason Rob was called for this particular liver was because we were only forty-five minutes from the hospital ... They were procuring the donor organ and needed someone to be worked up and ready to go within two hours. So moving to St. Augustine was the absolute best decision!

The role of caregiver after a transplant is a major part of the whole deal. That is why I am allowed to be here, because they are training me. It is a twenty-four-hour job. Thankfully, my brother drove down to help with Skye. Tonight, seeing each other for the first time since the transplant, she ran to me in front of the hospital like she hadn't seen me in a month. They will not let her come up to see Rob, so we had a picnic on the beautiful Mayo Clinic grounds.

Caregivers are responsible for keeping track of all important anti-rejection and other medications. They gave me a binder, and I have to record everything and report back to them. When we leave the hospital, we must regularly take his temperature, and if it's even a point higher than normal, go to the hospital immediately. He may also have to have his blood sugar monitored because many transplant patients have short-term diabetes when they take prednisone.

Dr. Mao sent us the pictures of Rob's old liver after they took it out and the new liver inside him before they closed him up. (When posting these on Facebook, we warned: "If you are squeamish, don't look. We, however, think the human body inside and out is incredibly amazing. The more we see, the more we know.")

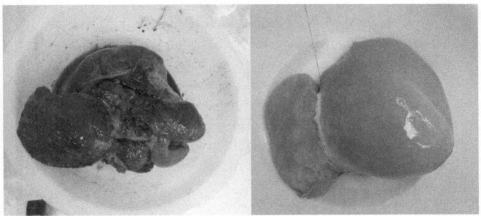

Rob's old liver   Rob's new liver
(Visit www.lezlee.com for color photos)

We did our weekly Friday Zoom session from the hospital with some of our local transplant friends Ron, Jerry, Gloria (Andy's wife), Alicia, and John. Now that Rob is on the other side, I had so many questions for them, and they were so helpful!

They told us that the steroids could make Rob have mood swings. He may cry easier or get angry. I prefer crying.

I got to see his wound stitching in the shape of a beautiful peace sign logo.

Rob will stay in the hospital until Monday or Tuesday, then come back three times a week. After a month or so, we leave and come back three months later and then only once a year.

There is a thirty percent chance that Rob could get PSC again because it is an autoimmune disorder. That would be terrible. But that also means there is a seventy percent chance that PSC won't return!

————•————

September 12, Day 3

Last night, I actually went into a real deep sleep, something I had not done in the prior forty-eight hours. This morning, a nurse came in to give Rob his medication. I was supposed to write everything down in the logbook, but I could not move. She asked me if I wanted her to do it, and I gratefully said "yes!"

The main goal for today is to get Rob's bowels moving again. That's right. If he toots or poops, that means they can take the tube out of his nose. It is not a feeding tube but is pulling bile from his stomach. Many PSC transplant patients have their whole bile duct taken out during surgery, and a surgical biliary reconstruction procedure is done, which requires the tube. If the tube can come out, he can begin ingesting clear liquids.

Every Mayo Clinic employee is so incredibly professional and pays such attention to detail. It is a well-oiled machine, which gives us confidence in the care. Even with such a serious surgery, there is a level of great calm here.

Rob's daytime nurse today, Deb, is so informative. I ask a *lot* of questions, especially to people who have been here for twenty years, like her. Everyone on this floor has had either a liver, kidney, or pancreas transplant. Deb explained that some of the most important life-saving factors today are the anti-rejection medications taken afterwards. I did not realize that the hepatologists custom-prepare drug therapy for each patient depending on their blood work. Most drugs are taken at 8 a.m. and 8 p.m. every day. Missing a dose could be tragic.

Rob pulled himself up and even used the walker independently today. He could barely move yesterday. We joke around and even play doctor (not what you're thinking). He starts directing me as only a captain does, which annoys me but makes me smile because I know he is coming back to life. His OCD is kicking in. He likes the surface of his tray table clear except for the necessities.

Saturdays at Mayo are quiet. Weekdays are hopping. The cafe and gift shop are closed today. Since all of this has happened, I have not taken a moment to reflect or even feel. Instead, I have been on autopilot, turning off my emotions, and remaining "strong" doing what I have to do.

But today, I am alone, walking around the grounds letting it all in. It is peaceful. I let myself feel and breathe. I think about Rob opening his eyes regaining consciousness, looking over to me and saying, "I love you, Lez. Thank you for sticking by me." He hasn't always been that vocal. This damn disease created an angry man who often withheld affection to "protect me."

The strangest cry I have ever heard suddenly erupts from my mouth, almost like a howling. Hugging a tree with Spanish moss dripping from it, I thank Mom. I thank God. I thank all the people who have prayed for us for so many days. I even thank the pain and the anger so I can feel the happiness and gratitude. And then it starts raining.

As soon as I enter room 317, the nurse is pulling out the tube, and Rob looks like Rob again!

We are now watching a movie together. It feels like a normal night ... except we are in a hospital room, and he has another person's major organ inside of him keeping him alive while the drugs are suppressing his immune system so his body won't reject it.

Skye just Facetimed me wearing my pajamas and sleeping in our bed on "Daddy's side" because she misses us.

———•———

September 13, Day 4

9 a.m.: All night long, they were taking blood from Rob and found out his liver counts are higher than usual. So they just brought

a whole ultrasound machine into the room, and Dr. Croome, one of the head liver transplant surgeons, and the PA have just come in to look at the pictures of Rob's liver. They need to rule out things like vascular obstruction of the bile duct.

The duct looks good, but they want to bring him downstairs for another procedure called a cholangiogram where they shoot dye into it. Thank goodness, when that's done, it shows there is no blockage.

Instead, he is having normal rejection, which they can control by giving him more steroids. Never a dull moment!

10 a.m.: I make a little video of nurse Deb explaining the importance of transplant drugs.

We are thankful to have made such good friends here through our support group, who are assuring us that all of the anti-rejection is to be expected.

11 a.m.: Needing a light moment, I videotape myself singing my song "Be a Giver of Your Liver." Nurse Deb loves it and is dancing in the background while Rob is holding up his blue Mayo Clinic pillow in the shape of a liver! I send it to Skye and River. All they have known is a mother who breaks into song at any moment. This is totally normal to them. They don't even question it. LOL.

12:10 p.m.: Our friend Jerry, who was the first person I interviewed for my book, wants to have lunch with me so he picks me up, and we go to the Crab Shack. Then he drives me to look at a few nearby marinas where we may move our tugboat so we can stay on it when we come back to Mayo in the future.

5 p.m.: Scott took Skye to the Jacksonville Zoo, and then he picks me up. We three go to this fun "escape room" where we have to find clues to open locks to the next phase. We wear our masks, wash hands, and are the only ones in the room.

7 p.m.: Sunday night's lobby at Mayo Clinic is practically empty except the man cleaning the floor and one security guard. Skye, Scott, and I eat our Chinese food in the fancy lobby, then I hug them goodbye before Scott will drive Skye back to St. Augustine. As

we were walking, she asked me, "Is Daddy going to be active again like when I was three?"

I am now resting beside Rob. He may have to have a liver biopsy tomorrow depending on the levels. This will be an up-and-down process.

September 14, Day 5

Notes from the morning:

- Nurses come in to take vitals and administer medication. Rob shows me his eyes, and they are a little yellow again. Damn it! What does that mean?
- I go downstairs to the main lobby and enjoy seeing activity, as people are coming for outpatient services. The Bundy Cafe is open, so I get some breakfast with a cup of hazelnut coffee and sit outside at one of the umbrella tables.
- I spot our surgeons, Dr. Mao and Dr. Croome, in the lobby and ask them about Rob's high liver enzyme levels causing jaundice. They tell me he is going for a biopsy and not to worry. If it is rejection, then they increase the steroids. But he is not ready to go home until they know. I feel confident.
- When I come back to the room, two residents are pulling out a tube from Rob's stomach while he grimaces. Not fun.

Notes from mid-day:

- They wheel Rob off to get his biopsy. He comes back, and I take an hour-long "caregivers" online class with a slide show.
- At 2 p.m., one of the nurses gives a thorough review of the medicines and what we need to know upon discharge. My head is spinning from all this information.
- Rob will never be able to eat grapefruit or orange marmalade (not that he ever did). If he is at a restaurant, he cannot eat raw vegetables at all or go to a buffet. All food has to be thoroughly

cooked, and fruits and veggies need to be run under water one full minute.

- He will be on a drug called Prograf for the rest of his life. He has to take it exactly twelve hours apart, 8 a.m. and 8 p.m. This is his most important anti-rejection drug, which lowers his immune response so the body doesn't attack the foreign liver. Other drugs get tapered off or added. He takes antiviral drugs too.

- If he ever has a headache that won't go away, feels sick at all, sees stars, or has a temperature of 99, we are to call Mayo immediately. This means he either has too much or too little Prograf in his system. What could be a normal cold for us is different for transplant recipients. You can never be too careful.

- Being around dogs is okay but not reptiles or even animals that eat their own poop. Our beloved guinea pig, Mishi, will have to be limited to Skye's room. The gecko has to go.

- No gardening with hands in the dirt or working on engines.

- More prone to skin cancer now, Rob must wear sunscreen all the time and stay covered.

- He has to wear a mask at all times, even when driving in the car, because of the recycled air and must stay six feet away from people. Hmmm. What does that sound like?

Notes from late afternoon and evening:

- We get a call from one of the staff members about the results of Rob's biopsy. He has something called moderate preservation injury; the donor liver was slightly injured while it was on ice, but it will repair itself on its own. There is no need for any outside intervention. This is not uncommon but happens more with kidneys.

- I sing the "Be a Giver of Your Liver" song to the nurses on call, and they, too, do background dancing, then call others down the hall to hear it. Maybe this could be a theme song!

- Rob orders an actual meal for the first time.
- I decide to take the advice on "self-care" from my caregiver class. Scott picks me up, and we drive back to St. Augustine so I can take a proper shower and spend the night in a real bed.

September 15, Day 6

Notes from the morning:

- I get to Rob's hospital room just before the weekly Mayo Clinic Second Chance Support Group Zoom meeting at 11 a.m. There are about thirty people from all over the country, who are either pre- or post-transplant. Today, Rob gives the most emotional speech (which is recorded) telling them he has finally gotten his transplant. At the end, with his voice cracking, he says, "You gotta hold on. Don't give up. You gotta hold on!"
- Dr. Yang, hepatologist, and Dr. Mao come to the room and ask Rob if he feels strong enough to go home today. What? We are shocked. Rob says he wants to practice walking up some stairs but other than that he feels good enough!

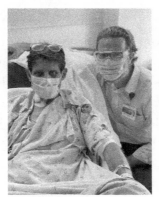

Rob with Mike Womack

Notes from mid-day:

- Social worker and friend Mike Womack comes to visit Rob in full mask like everyone because of COVID.
- Science writer Lara Pullen emails me to let me know that the editor of *The American Journal of Transplantation* wants her to write an article based on the petition I put together asking for exception points on MELD scores for PSC patients! It will be featured in the December issue. I cannot believe it.
- One of the nurses comes to give us a lesson on taking Rob's glucose levels, which often rise when taking steroids after transplant. If the level is over 140, insulin must be given. We get the whole kit and practice giving a shot, which we will have to do that evening.

Notes from late afternoon and evening:

- The liver coordinator goes over all the medication and presents us with a special Mayo Clinic briefcase with shoulder bag where we will keep all our meds and binder. Rob is extremely independent and used to taking all his meds on his own from years of having PSC. Letting me be part of it will be challenging for him, but nurses tell him he has to let me assist.
- We load up everything, and Rob gets wheeled downstairs while I get the car. He jokingly asks for a sedative while I drive! I make him go in the back seat. He's back!
- We park in front of our St. Augustine condo. Scott and Skye come down to help with bags. Rob slowly gets out of the car. Skye hugs her daddy while he lifts up his shirt and shows off his scar. Wearing her colorful circus hat, she takes him by the hand and leads him to the entrance, which is decorated with streamers and balloons. Our neighbors, Heidi and Kit, helped her decorate. Rob climbs the stairs with no difficulty. Another neighbor, Angie, brings food she has made.
- Rob takes a nice hot shower and shaves.

- We display all of his drugs out on the kitchen table ready to organize. Rob takes his pills, and I write it down in the log. Then we have to figure out the glucose insulin kit, which was slightly complicated, but we did it! Rob's sugar was 226 so he needed six units of insulin.
- Eyes heavy. Brain fried. We need to be at the hospital by 7:30 a.m. for Rob to give blood, then take his medication at 8 a.m.

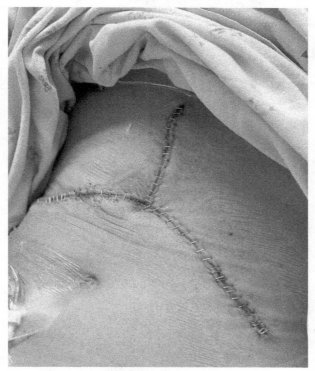

First look at staples

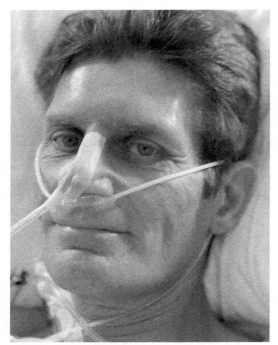

First smile

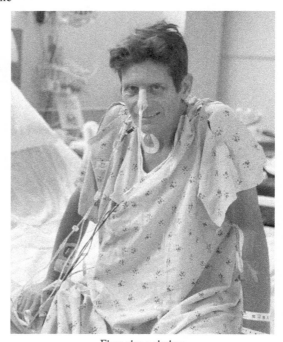

First time sitting

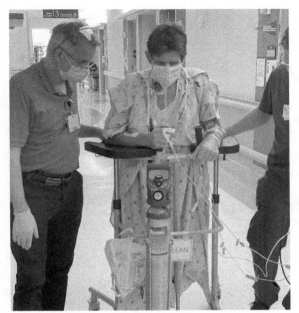

First walk

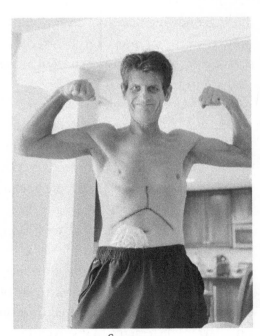

Superman

CHAPTER 35

Dr. Shennen Mao: From Pig Farmer to Liver Transplant Surgeon

When Dr. Shennen Mao introduced herself to us before the surgery, my first impression was that while she might be relatively young, her self-confidence and steady speech gave us a safe feeling, knowing that Rob's liver would be in her hands. Our instincts were correct. She proved to be excellent not only in performing the transplant, but also in her thorough communication with us before and afterwards.

Dr. Mao, who graduated from Harvard Medical School in 2009, was only thirty-seven years old when she performed Rob's transplant on September 10, 2020. One of two women among the six abdominal transplant surgeons at Mayo Clinic in Jacksonville, she led a surgical team of eight people, including six female and two male professionals, who went back and forth between two simultaneous liver transplant surgeries that were being performed in rooms near each other.

Dr. Mao grew up on the same pig farm where her father had grown up, outside a tiny Iowa town of 402 people north of Des Moines. Both her parents shared in running the farm. "Growing up on a farm, you're actively involved in everything that's going on, so

I always say that I've given more shots to pigs than I ever will to people," she joked.

Originally, she thought she would be a veterinarian. Watching the vets who traveled from farm to farm, she began to pick up some basic skills. "My parents and I were soon able to tell if something was wrong with one of our animals. Since then, I have always had an interest in the sciences," she said.

"In high school, I worked as a nursing assistant at a local nursing home and realized that I liked talking to people because they could tell me what was wrong with them, as opposed to an animal where you have to potentially guess. So, after that, I decided I wanted to go to medical school."

She attended Creighton University, a Jesuit Catholic university in Omaha, Nebraska, where she played trumpet, took numerous music classes, and had a biology and chemistry double major. There, she also met the young man who later became her husband, Dr. Michael Mao. After going on to complete medical school, both she and Michael did their residency at Mayo Clinic in Rochester, Minnesota. He is now a general nephrologist at Mayo Clinic in Jacksonville, treating acute kidney failure as well as kidney injuries and disease.

In the middle of her five-year residency, she did a two-year research fellowship with a liver transplant surgeon in Rochester, Dr. Scott Nyberg. She completed her seven-year residency/fellowship in 2016.

Part of her fellowship research involved developing a liver support device similar to kidney dialysis. "When a patient has liver disease, a lot of supportive care is needed. One of the questions we ask is: Can we help patients with liver disease, especially acute liver disease, clear the toxins in their blood better with a machine?" Dr. Mao said.

"In the experiment, only pigs were used, not humans, but the concept was the same," she explained. The animal's liver cells came into contact with the liver-diseased blood from another pig, and then the blood was cleared and given back to the "pig patient." She pointed out that many research facilities use pigs, as the animal's anatomy is similar to that of a human, especially the size of the liver.

"One of the big things that happens in humans is that they get too sick for transplant," Dr. Mao said. "The question is, can a device help support that patient until a liver becomes available? When I looked for a lab, using pigs was a perk to me since I was familiar with this species, and it was a perk to the lab to have someone who knew about pigs as well."

The lab model was successful, but the experiments have not yet been done in humans. The team in Rochester is still working on getting FDA approval, and Dr. Mao currently is working on other transplant-related projects in labs at Mayo Clinic Jacksonville as well. "Doing transplants on pigs is not the same as humans," she commented. "But it is very similar. I certainly gained operative exposure with these animals that influenced my future practice."

She was honored in 2018 that she could remain at Mayo after her fellowship, when the job became available as a transplant surgeon. "You are never left alone, always learning, and gaining experience," she said. "That is what is particularly wonderful about Mayo Clinic Transplant. We have a great group of abdominal surgeons. If there is ever a time when anyone needs assistance in the operating room, we can pick up the phone and call. All of us live within ten to fifteen minutes away.

"The night that I did your husband's surgery, I was on call for kidney transplant. My colleague, Dr. Croome, was on call for liver transplant. Whoever is on call for that organ makes the decision on who the recipient will be. We happened to get a second liver offer at the same time, which is rare, and Dr. Croome asked if I would come and put the liver in your husband. I said, absolutely!"

The hospital does only fifteen to twenty pancreas transplants a year. "The big rarity with those is the donor," Dr. Mao said. "This particular organ is susceptible to injury, and as we get older, it becomes infiltrated with fat, particularly with the American diet, so the likelihood of it being a good pancreas is lower. In liver transplants, you can use an eighty-year-old liver, and it is probably okay."

She explained that the most common form of liver cancer is hepatocellular carcinoma (HCC). A patient with HCC could receive a transplant, provided the tumors did not exceed a certain size and number, and provided the cancer had not spread beyond the liver.

"If we had enough readily available organs, we would transplant everyone," she said. "But we don't want to give an organ to someone with aggressive cancer who is likely to end up dying a year after transplant, when the organ could have benefited someone else. Unfortunately, we have to make hard choices about allocating a rare resource."

People with Rob's disease, PSC, would more likely develop bile duct cancer, or cholangiocarcinoma, Dr. Mao explained. It spreads and acts differently from an HCC, as cholangiocarcinoma typically travels in the bile duct, so it potentially can grow into the pancreas. After learning this, Rob and I were even more grateful that he had been able to get his transplant now, before bile duct cancer could develop.

"In terms of liver diseases, we see a lot more people in this country with non-alcoholic steatohepatitis, which is certainly related to the American diet causing fatty liver and obesity. It stems probably from both the types and quantities of food," Dr. Mao pointed out.

Discussing MELD scores, she said, "The MELD score is probably the most objective way that we have to allocate a very sparse resource. Unfortunately, MELD scores cannot capture everything. It is objective, in taking a set of laboratory values and using them to assign a score. The score is not perfect, and while I do not think we should put things in the score that are subjective, some people are sicker than what their score indicates. We, as a transplant community, are obligated to continually evaluate our system and to look at groups of patients to see how we can serve them better."

She added, "The biggest thing we can do is advocate for more people to sign up to be donors. We are trying, as a transplant center, to use more marginal donors—meaning donors who are older, whose livers have more fat, and using special preservation devices that can prolong donor liver viability."

Unfortunately, much misconception and wrong information leads people to be scared of signing up to be an organ donor, thinking the medical community will not do everything possible to save their life if they are injured.

"If we knew where that misconception came from, we would combat it one hundred percent," Dr. Mao said. "The procurement team is not even notified until the patient is declared legally brain-dead or, in the case of a cardiac death donor, when the family has requested the withdrawal of life-sustaining measures. There could be a potential donor in my own hospital, and I'd have no knowledge of that individual."

Once the transplant center has a suitable organ, the on-call surgeon has the responsibility of matching the organ to the recipient, and there is not a lot of time to do so. "Essentially, you start at the top of the transplant list," she said, "and you try to put the organ into the first person you have who is appropriate."

While a higher MELD score is the most significant factor, size of the donated organ also makes a difference. "You cannot put a larger liver into a smaller-sized person, but you could put a smaller one into a larger person because livers grow," Dr. Mao explained. In Rob's case, his PSC disease had increased the size of his liver and stretched out his rib cage, even though he is not a particularly large man, which meant that a bigger liver could be used.

"One of the reasons, in fact, that Rob received the liver he did was because the original recipient was too small," she said. "There is research indicating that smaller people, women in particular, are somewhat disadvantaged because of their frame size. And while men tend to be taller, that does not mean that we only put male livers in male recipients. Liver size typically correlates to the person's height, but not always; we like to get a CT scan of the donor, so we can physically measure the liver. It is about size, not gender, and race does not matter either."

Before any recovery of organs takes place, the organ procurement coordinators must do a lot of testing including HIV, hepatitis, COVID, and additional heart and lung testing. This could take hours or even days.

"Part of being a transplant surgeon requires doing organ recovery from a deceased donor," Dr. Mao said. "I have always tried to think about it as a way to honor the dying wishes of a patient or their family member and a way of extending the care of that patient beyond their death. I also look at it as an opportunity to hopefully make a positive impact out of a tragedy, knowing that the family members are going through what is the worst day of their life. Perhaps I can help a bit by bringing hope and new life to multiple recipients on the other end."

A practicing Christian, she feels that her faith does influence her role as a transplant surgeon. "In our field, we deal with a larger than average amount of death and loss in our donor families. Before each procurement, I always share a small private prayer for the donor prior to beginning the operation."

There is always a risk of death with this type of surgery, she noted. "However, liver transplant at our center is associated with lower than one percent intraoperative mortality, and the one-year survival rate is ninety-four percent."

Dr. Mao gave birth to her son, Xavier, in March 2020 and had continued doing transplants up to the end of her pregnancy. "I've always been an individual who has a lot of energy and does not need a lot of sleep," she chuckled.

Asked how she sees her future, she said, "I get a lot of joy from clinical work, so I hope that I am still transplanting patients and affecting individual lives. On the research side, I hope I've been able to affect some aspects of transplant reaching more patients. Clinically, I can realistically take care of seven or eight patients a week. In the research lab, I'd hope to help make discoveries and developments that would affect hundreds of patients.

"I love my job. I love the values that Mayo Clinic puts forward so I don't see myself leaving here anytime soon."

Rob, who is particularly happy with the meticulous scar left from Dr. Mao's incision, is extremely thankful she was his surgeon. This doctor walked into our hospital room as a stranger who matched and put the precious organ of another stranger inside my husband, saving his life. What a miracle.

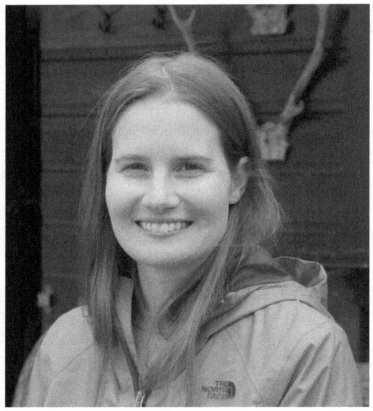

Dr. Shennen Mao

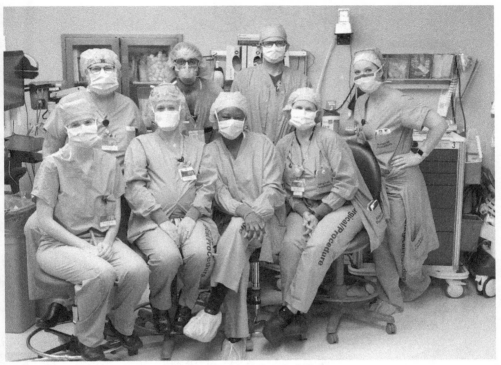

Rob's Transplant Surgical Team
Back row (L to R): Cheryl Thompson, PAC (surgical first assistant), Ryan Chad-
ha, MD (staff anesthesiologist), Peter Davis (perfusion), Brittany Blake, APRN,
CRNA, DNP (anesthesia). Front row (L to R): Shennen Mao, MD (staff surgeon),
Haley Hawkinberry, MSN, RN (OR circulating nurse), Marie Holloman (surgical
technologist), Shauna Jackson, RN (OR circulating nurse)

CHAPTER 36

Celebrating One Week After Transplant!

September 16, 2020, St. Augustine and Jacksonville

Mayo Clinic puts transplant patients on a rigorous schedule after they are released because they need to constantly check blood work and adjust medication.

- 6 a.m.: Scott leaves for Atlanta, so Skye decides she wants to come with us to our first all-day appointments at Mayo Clinic. I figure she can just do online school in one of the sitting areas using their Wi-Fi. I usually drive Mom's old Prius, but Rob wants to take his Mercedes SUV because the ride is more comfortable. The problem is that I haven't had a lot of experience driving his fancy car with all the bells and whistles. Needless to say, Rob was a nervous wreck in the back seat while I almost stripped the gears by accident. Having him direct my every move didn't help. I asked if he could have an OCD transplant as well. We got to the Davis Building in time for the 6:30 a.m. ultrasound of his liver.

- 7:40 a.m.: Blood work, pills, breakfast

- 8 a.m.: Skye cannot get on the Mayo Clinic Wi-Fi at all. Computer crashes. I call the school and explain the situation. They say, "Do *not* worry!" I figure she will learn more on that day than otherwise.

- 9:30 a.m.: Having some time to kill, we take the Mercedes to the dealer to get an oil change. Everyone has masks on, and Rob wants to check out the showroom. He decides to display his Mercedes-logo-shaped incision, and the salespeople are blown away and start taking pictures. We ask if we put a circle around it, could we get a huge discount? You never know.

- 12:30 p.m.: We head back to Mayo for the next appointment. I miss the turn and basically realize that I am way too intimidated to drive this car and prefer a plain ol' regular car. Rob is getting more pissed off, which makes me drive worse. I finally find a parking space after much searching but forget to put it in park. That's it. Rob can't take it anymore. He says he is driving, no matter what. I can't stop laughing.

- 1:15 p.m.: We meet with one of the post-transplant nurses, Adam, who looks at Rob's blood work and wound and says it looks really good. Skye has to stay in the lobby.

- 2:45 p.m.: We rush down to the cafe to eat a sandwich. But first, Rob uses the glucose kit to check his blood sugar. The steroids create a "fight or flight," which raises the level. Sure enough, it is over 140, so he gives himself two units.

- 4 p.m.: We go back upstairs for the next appointment. A woman recognizes me as I am lying down on one of the long seats. We realize that our husbands had their liver transplants on the *same* day at the *same* time with the *same* blood type! Twin liver transplant recipients! Naturally, we take a picture with Rob and Eddie lifting up their shirts to display their scars.

- 5 p.m.: We meet with one of the hepatologists, Dr. Raj, who says he wants us to increase Rob's level of Prograf to get the liver count level down. That means we have to come back on Saturday at 7:40 a.m. to do blood work again so he can check levels. It is all about the tweaking. The woman at the scheduling desk compliments me on how well-behaved Skye has been waiting patiently for us.

- 6:30 p.m.: We drive back to St Augustine. I won't say who did the driving, but it was a good driver. We stop at a nice seafood restaurant in Ponte Vedra and get a table outside. We talk to the owner and say we are celebrating something special. Then Skye blurts out, "My daddy had a liver transplant." The owner is so happy to hear this and sends a "congratulations" key lime pie after dinner, which I did not intend to need to eat, but do.

- 8:30 p.m.: Both of us are beyond exhausted but have to go over his meds and record them in the book.

- 9 p.m.: My stomach hurts, and I am bending over, but then Rob needs my help putting a pillow behind his head. OMG, we feel like we are elderly people!

While it would be nice to think we will just walk into the sunset, and life will become blissfully perfect, we all know that is impossible. Normal life is filled with twists, turns, unexpected highs, and lows. Right now, what we can hope for is that the worst of this health crisis is behind us.

—————•—————

Monday, September 17

We leave the condo at 6:45 a.m. to go back to Mayo Clinic for continued monitoring.

Rob did not think he needed his walker today, but the Mayo campus is large, so he now leans on me while we walk together into the Cannaday Building where he gets his blood drawn. It feels nice knowing he needs to hold onto me for support—both physically and emotionally. We run into one of our support group friends, Lynn, and her husband, David. Lynn is here for her yearly checkup. She had her transplant on September 11, 2017.

After pills and breakfast, we meet with Kim, our new liver transplant coordinator. She tells us that Rob's blood work numbers are "trending in the right direction," and that is a good thing, but our meeting with the hepatologist at 2:45 will tell us more.

We go downstairs, and Rob takes an extra-strength Tylenol for back pain. We have about an hour to kill, so I encourage him to come out to the scenic grounds in front of my favorite moving windmill statue in the pond. We make it to a bench, and Rob lies down on my lap while I begin reading excerpts from a wonderful life-affirming book, *Tuesdays with Morrie*. I can't help but make the comparison of "Tuesdays with Support Group." There is a pleasant breeze, and Rob falls into a deep sleep. I feel bad waking him up, but we need to get to the last appointment for the day.

While we are in the lobby, Rob asks if I could please not ask a bunch of questions so we can get in and out of there because he is tired. No problem. It should be a quick visit.

Just before our meeting with Dr. Raj, hepatologist, the nurse tells us that Dr. Mao is meeting with us too. Hmmm. That seems a little odd but whatever.

Dr. Raj, a jovial man who studied in India, takes a look at Rob's stitches, goes over the blood work, and then pulls out a yellow pad and begins drawing a picture of the liver, bile duct, stomach, and pancreas. As he is talking, I realize that I better pay attention and maybe even videotape so I can refer back later.

He explains that when doctors take out a patient's old liver, it gets sent to pathology for further analysis. I was wondering what they do with it and happy it wasn't thrown out in the trash because it was so ugly! Anyway, Dr. Raj tells us that there was some "high-grade dysplasia" on the old bile duct and along the cut, which did not show up in the MRI.

Dysplasia is a broad term that refers to the abnormal development of cells within tissues or organs. It can lead to a wide range of conditions involving enlarged tissue or precancerous cells.

Apparently, there was much discussion over the weekend with people from Mayo Clinic in Rochester about Rob and "what to do" if anything. Next thing I know, Dr. Mao walks in, and using the picture that Dr. Raj drew, she explains more clearly the *Roux-en-Y* procedure has re-routed the bile from the liver, and his remaining bile duct, which leads to the pancreas, is essentially just "sitting there" doing nothing.

Many PSC patients are prone to bile duct cancer, so you want to get the transplant done before this happens, which is why I am so adamant that UNOS give exception points on MELD scores to avoid this. The longer the patient is on the waitlist, the more their chances are of getting a carcinoma. Let's be clear. Rob does *not* have cancer. But there is this high-grade dysplasia along where she cut and possibly farther down. She needed us to know that this is very rare and that they don't quite know what the best course of action is. Wow! Have we really stumped the Mayo Clinic?

She and Dr. Raj give us the options:

1. Do nothing right now except "surveillance," watching it carefully with CT scans and an endoscopy in four months. It is a little challenging because you can't get in there anymore with a scope.

2. Burn off the area somehow—but we would have to go to Mayo in Rochester to do this.

3. The most radical thing would be for Rob to have another surgery, five or more hours. Dr. Mao would open up the same incision and get rid of that dysplasia. However, if it continued to show dysplasia farther down the bile duct, she might have to do one of the biggest surgeries there—a "Whipple procedure" to remove the head of the pancreas, the first part of the small intestine (duodenum), the gallbladder, and the bile duct.

Whaaaaat???!! Are you kidding me? Rob doesn't even panic or pause.

"Surveillance," he says definitively. "Let's just watch it. The biggest hurdle is over with. I do not want to risk my life again when I have precancerous cells that could lead to nothing. If there is no bile going in there, then my chance of getting cancer is much lower."

I ask Dr. Mao what she would do if this was her husband, and she says to keep a close eye on it. She explains all the possible things that could happen with another surgery, and it just seems too much. Rob has been through enough. Let him heal.

Driving back, we are in disbelief. We thought it would be a normal visit. You never know what is around the corner.

Bottom line: The Mayo Clinic looks at everything. This hiccup was out of the ordinary, and they wanted us to have all the information.

Realizations from the Transplant World:

If just one person decides to sign up to be an organ donor from all of these details, I will have done my job. That is how I truly feel. I don't believe in privacy when it comes to this subject because it is too important.

We are literally all the same underneath, and there is no way to tell a "female" liver from a "male" liver or what color, religion, sexual-orientation, socio-economic, or political affiliation the person who donated was. It is simply a healthy organ or not. No one can afford to discriminate, and so there is simply a gratitude and appreciation that you feel from a transplant recipient.

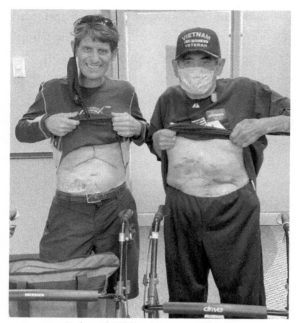

Rob and Eddie showing off scars

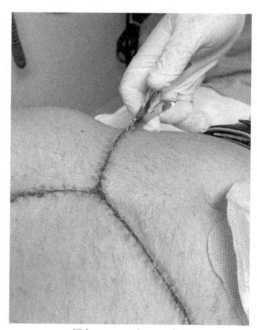

Taking out the staples

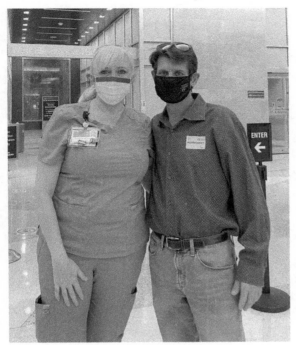

Rob with Nurse Deb

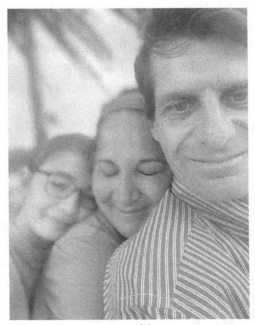

Grateful

CHAPTER 37

Reflections from Captain Rob

October 2020

Several weeks after Rob's transplant, my uncle Roy, a seasoned writer, came from Alabama to visit us. He had read some early chapters from my book and offered to interview Rob and gather his perspectives about the experience.

After talking a little about the long, wearing months before the transplant, Roy asked how he had felt when he woke up after the surgery and realized it was done.

"The first thing I noticed was the olive-colored wallpaper in front of me and realized I could see color again," Rob said. "Before the transplant, I could not see the beauty of life in the world. We would be sitting outside on the deck of this condo looking at the palm trees. The colors were dull, but when I woke up, I was so happy to be alive. I was reenergized, feeling like I had a new engine inside me ready to roll!

"Everyone in the support group had kept telling me to look at myself in the mirror afterwards," he recalled. "My color was coming back to normal; the whites of my eyes were not yellow anymore right after surgery. I was determined to get up and walk as soon as possible, and my body began to recover fairly quickly."

As they sat on the condo's balcony overlooking the water, Roy asked, "What do you see from here that you didn't see before September 10?"

"I see life, color, and light. I see the second chance that I have, but I'm cautious because you don't know how your body will react to the new liver and the medication," Rob replied. "I want to move forward in a different direction in life. I'm worried about the stress, the business, and the environment of New York. It makes you have a thick coat of hardness. Up north, I feel like it's hard to focus on enjoying life because it's so expensive, and there's always so much to do to keep up with the high cost of living. It's not something I'm looking forward to going back to."

He pointed out that at Mayo and with the support group, "It's like you are being born again. Mayo is like your mother. And you are her little duckling, and you don't want to leave your mother. I will continue to do the weekly Zoom meetings with the support group. It's not only the environment, but I have gotten such amazing care at Mayo Clinic. I am probably having separation anxiety."

There were positives about the year in St. Augustine, despite his illness, the fears, and the quarantine, he said. "It has been great that I've been able to spend all of this time with my family. I have experienced life outside of business, and I don't want my life to be about how much I can accumulate before I retire."

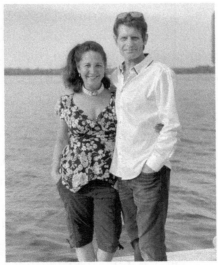

Lezlee and Rob, six weeks post-transplant

CHAPTER 38

Mike: The Social Worker's Perspective

How could I not include a chapter from our cherished support group leader, Michael Womack, whose voice we look forward to hearing every week?

"I am not rich monetarily," Mike admitted. "But I am certainly rich in perspective. Working with so many transplant patients, one common theme is appreciation. Finding out what you really need in life and appreciating what you have is so important."

He became the facilitator of the Second Chance Support Group for kidney, liver, and pancreas transplants in 2010, a few months before he was officially hired as a Mayo Clinic social worker. Patients and caregivers who are on the transplant list or who already have had transplants know that every Tuesday at 11 a.m. is the time to gather to share updates, ask questions, and feel connected with those who are in the same situation.

"I like the dialogue, I like the participation, I like the stories," Mike told me. "It's not my group. I am there to keep it in play and let it evolve without an agenda unless something specific has happened. This allows participants to get what they need to get out of it. Even when hearing the same stories over and over, something new and different comes out each week."

One unexpected outcome from the pandemic of 2020 was that

instead of temporarily shutting down the support group, Mike continued the weekly meetings via Zoom. This expanded the group from an average of fifteen people locally to an average of more than thirty online. They provide input from their homes in different states where they would otherwise be unable to.

"I think accessibility to anything, especially in health care, is key to even better care," Mike asserted. "At Mayo, anything to better the experience of patient care is a good thing."

Born in Annapolis, Maryland, in 1981, Mike described himself as a "military brat without moving around a lot." His father was a fighter pilot in Vietnam and a Naval Academy graduate, and Mike and his two brothers grew up near Pensacola, Florida. His mother raised the children and returned to being an art and preschool teacher. His parents divorced amicably when Mike was ten years old.

He began college in 1999 at the University of Central Florida in Orlando. "I didn't really do well at first and wasn't in the mind frame for school," Mike admitted. "So I went home to Pensacola for a couple of years to get myself together." He reenrolled at the University of West Florida in Pensacola in 2001 at age twenty-two and received his bachelor's degree in interdisciplinary social sciences four years later.

"Many people in life are late bloomers," he said with a smile, "and I must be one of them." While it took him longer than he expected to get his college diploma, master's degree in social work, and subsequent license, it was worth the patience and hard work.

"My original goal was to be a history teacher, but sometimes it takes a special person to see potential that you might not see in yourself. As an interdisciplinary science major, I had to take a social work class, and the professor told me she thought I would be great in this field. She spent extra time with me setting out a course path."

After graduating from UWF, Mike began working with Family First Network, a contractor for the Department of Children and Family Services, where he was a family services counselor visiting the kids in their homes and working with parents fulfilling whatever they needed to do for the court. At first it was interesting, but he quickly learned that this kind of work did not make him happy. "It felt like wandering around in the dark, then touching something and knowing you don't like that," Mike said.

He kept in touch with his social work professor, who continued to encourage him to get his master's degree. Suddenly more mature and focused, he completed a second bachelor's degree in social work in one semester at Florida State University, which then put him in an accelerated graduate school program, and he received his master's degree in 2009. "I immersed myself into their program at FSU and enjoyed it," Mike told me. "It is by far the top social work program in the Southeast. You are learning about social and human theory on a micro and macro level. I took more of a clinical track studying human behavior and psychology instead of policy making. I've always been a people person and wanted to work with individuals.

"In the spring before graduating, I wondered what I was going to do with this degree. I heard about a program offered by the U.S. Navy where, if accepted, they would send me somewhere to get my licensed clinical social worker certification. So I really applied myself and got accepted into this specialized officer training program. They had two options for me to get my supervision after graduation— either John Hopkins University in Baltimore or Mayo Clinic in Jacksonville. I had a choice, but they would ultimately decide for me. Being a beach boy my whole life fishing and boating, I wanted to stay in Florida. So, through the military, they sent me to the Mayo Clinic. By the way, this program with Mayo ran its course, so luck and timing were everything."

While working in various areas of the hospital, Mike started training under the liver transplant social worker, learning the role as it related to the transplant team. In mid-2010, that employee took a medical leave and then retired. "From May through July, I was doing the social worker job in this department. When I was hired as an official employee, I went back to work in that liver transplant role, which they needed, and obtained my license from the State of Florida in November 2011," Mike explained. "I got into the liver transplant department by chance but quickly became immersed and fulfilled in this role."

In 2012, Mike met his wife, Andi, a dietician, through social media. Ironically, he had graduated from high school with her sister but had not known Andi then. They now have two daughters.

Centers for Medicare and Medicaid Services (CMS) guidelines require that all potential transplant patients be seen by a social worker as part of their evaluation. The majority of Mike's job is assessing transplant readiness for patients with liver disease, determining whether they meet certain required criteria, and interfacing with them on their return visits.

The Mayo Clinic evaluates hundreds of patients yearly. At any given time, the transplant waiting list has an average of 100 people, though they could have been evaluated previously. Many people who are evaluated do not get on the transplant list right away for different reasons; for example, it may be too early in their disease, or they still need to relocate closer to the hospital. In the interim, the team follows them so that once they are ready, the team is ready.

The social worker has to establish important factors with potential patients. The first necessity is making sure that person has a caregiver with the proper support during and after transplant. Unfortunately, Mike has had to turn people away who did not have support, perhaps because they were estranged from family members, their family was deceased, or they had no one close to them to step up and help them. Sometimes, people can hire others to be caregivers.

Secondly, the patient has to have the ability to comply with the post-transplant regimen, such as getting the important medicine and taking it regularly, because this is a lifelong commitment.

Thirdly, while waiting, the person must live no more than six hours driving distance from the Mayo Clinic and then must stay in Jacksonville for a minimum amount of time after the surgery to make sure there is no rejection.

Mostly, the person has to want this and be motivated to do what needs to be done. Over the years, Mike has seen people who wanted to do it but did not have the ability, or who were only doing it because their spouse or children wanted them to. Some people realized after learning more about the procedure, they were simply too fearful or did not want to go through with it.

"You can sense ambivalence," he said. "To say no is a meaningful decision. As a social worker, you coach people towards the decision they want to make for themselves. I respect anyone who says yes or no. I have seen people decide that they have done everything they wanted to do in their life, did not want to risk the outcome of a surgery, or take away a younger person's opportunity of getting a transplant. Sometimes things happen so fast that they have not had time to process what is even happening."

Once a patient is accepted into the program, the same social worker usually follows them through their journey. At one point, Chaplain Services also facilitated the liver support group; then, Mike and another social worker shared the role of facilitator. Eventually, Mike became the only one leading the Tuesday group meetings.

"I like the energy and the people in the Second Chance group," he said, smiling. "I'm happy going to work knowing that I am helping people. Naturally, I develop a much closer bond with those who come to the group regularly, and they get to know me as well. I try to be real without a lot of technical language."

He continued, "You can't help but form attachments with transplant patients. There have definitely been people who have passed, and it hit me. What's great about the support group is that people come in at different phases—evaluation, the waiting period, and post-transplant. Everyone's stories are interesting, and they help each other. With life in general, you don't really know what you're going to get, you do the best you can, and nothing is guaranteed."

Mike has no interest in switching lanes from his area. "What I like about transplant is the humanity of it. Because of where the organs are coming from and the gift aspect of it, it is so precious. It is crazy to think that the part that you need is only made by another human biologically, not made in a factory somewhere, which makes it more real and requires more appreciation, which creates more personal responsibility. What is common is the appreciation for small things that become more important. My perspective of all of this is the best part of the job."

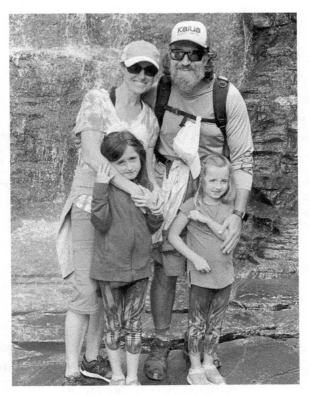

Mike Womack with his family

CHAPTER 39

Going Home to a Welcome Parade

Late October 2020, Florida to New York

Knowing that leaving St. Augustine with the safety of being near the Mayo Clinic was going to be difficult for Rob, I wanted to make his welcome home special. Many people in our hometown had been following our story through my Facebook posts. While folks may often shun social media, I have seen many positive outcomes from this platform, and I used it to organize a surprise parked-car parade for Rob on October 25, 2020, in Nyack.

Facebook had helped me reach a wide circle when we were looking for a living donor in 2018. An online PSC support group had helped Rob learn about the drug Vancomycin, which brought his liver counts down for a whole year before needing to be put on the transplant list.

In early October 2020, I had discovered the AlloCare Transplant Festival through Facebook and entered my song "Be a Giver of Your Liver," videotaped from the hospital with Rob and one of the nurses. Amazingly, the song won first place earning us $2,000.

The week before we left St. Augustine was spent with many socially distanced lunches, dinners, and goodbyes. Our friend Toosie and her husband, Dennis, hosted a fabulous lunch at her Ponte Vedra home with other support group friends, Andy, Gloria, Lynn, David, Jerry, and Alicia, attending.

Tim and Annie from the condo hosted a wonderful goodbye dinner with neighbors and friends, and Tim helped pull our ranger tugboat out of the water to store it at his cousin's storage yard. He said it would be no big deal to put it back in the water when we returned in January for Rob's four-month follow-up.

We had farewell outings with many other local friends, feeling loved and knowing we'd be missed.

As we pulled away from our condo, Rob's St. Augustine home for exactly one year—October 21, 2019, to October 21, 2020—I could feel the lump in my throat move up my face filling my eyes with tears. We did it! We accomplished our goal, and Rob was going home with a new working liver looking and feeling better every day.

We first drove to my brother Scott's house in Atlanta to see my father and rent a trailer to take home artwork and sentimental items from Mom that Scott had been storing. I told Dad that Rob had his liver transplant and it went well. He opened his eyes when Rob held my father's hands and showed him his scar. Scott went with us for the two-day drive back to Nyack.

My vision for the parade was to have people with signs stand along Midland Avenue, one of the main streets in town, before turning up one of the more private streets to our own. I had created a private Facebook event, put my friend Angela in charge, and asked people to make signs, stay in their car, and then pass by our house. I had also reached out to some local press.

Scott knew we had a 4 p.m. deadline, so we had to time the drive up perfectly. Rob kept asking if he could take over the driving, but Scott told him he was fine and to rest. I was driving the Prius, and they were behind me in the Mercedes SUV pulling the trailer.

Finally, we took the last exit on I-287 to Nyack and drove north along the familiar Midland Avenue. I was doing my very first "Facebook Live" from the car. At first, it looked like a normal fall day, and I wondered if anyone would even show up.

Suddenly, as we approached the street near our own, I saw a

cluster of people in their yard holding "Welcome Home Capt. Rob" signs, drumming, and waving, with a bonfire blazing. I beeped several times, rolled down the window, waved, and told them that Rob was right behind me. Skye slid down in her seat beside me, embarrassed as only a pre-teen could be. Scott opened the sunroof of the SUV, and once Rob realized the people were there cheering for him, he popped his head outside the top of the car and was overcome with emotion.

The farther down the street we went, the more people shouted, "Welcome home, Rob!" Several folks were even holding signs that read "Be a Giver of Your Liver," which made me shout with happiness. Then, we turned left up the hill leading to our street, and people with signs were sitting on top of their cars, cheering.

Finally, at the very top of the hill, our neighbor Lou shot off fireworks. *Fireworks* in Upper Nyack! I pulled into our driveway, got out, and watched Rob wiping tears of joy from his face.

Then, he spotted River in front of our home. He jumped out of the car and embraced his son, crying, "I didn't know if I would ever see you again."

There, on the side yard of our home, was a colorful sign put out by Anthony, a fellow veteran friend—saying "Welcome Home Capt. Rob," with a picture of Superman on one side and Wonder Woman on the other. My friend Cappi had inserted bright fall mums in our planters, and our friend Rich had decorated our front steps with pumpkins. I spotted so many of our friends like Jamie, Emily, Jon, Karim, Mike, Tiffany, Kevin, and Cynthia. Toni, Marty, and their kids were in tears and blowing kisses along with the Ehrenreich, Kapetonovic, Secklin, Sleebos and Shalom families. Carla was there wearing her familiar hat, worried people were getting too close because of Covid. I saw people cheering from my Nyack Bootcamp group, and then we held each other and stood in front of the driveway. People then drove by our home one by one to give Rob an individual greeting. It was one of the most exciting moments of our lives.

Later, I found out from another neighbor, who is not on Facebook and had no idea what was happening, that she was upset, knowing Rob was ill and fearing they were bringing his casket home! When she saw Rob waving from the SUV, she was so relieved.

Shortly after we came home, we drove to the nursing home where Rob's mother, Rosanna, had been living for more than a year. We gathered around but kept six feet apart in the outside entrance, and her face lit up when she saw her Rob. He lifted his shirt and showed her his scar. "I made it, Ma!" He smiled. She understood. Her son survived liver disease unlike her husband many years ago. Liver transplant had not been an option for Nino, and he died leaving her a widow with four sons. Life had come full circle.

Rob recently commented to a relative, "How is it that I can be one out of 170 liver transplant patients a year at the Mayo Clinic when there are thousands of people in the United States who are waiting for an organ? They do an average of two per week. We don't have enough donors in our country," he said.

"The fact that I received one is a miracle. Lezlee and I have more of a purpose in life to help others by promoting donation. Before going through this, I took life for granted. No one thinks about when their time is up unless you're faced with mortality in front of you. It changes you."

This was a chance at a new beginning for all of us, but what would "back to normal" feel like, especially in a pandemic that had virtually shut down our business and our whole way of socializing? We were coming back to bone-chilling cold with 4 p.m. darkness and an uncertain future.

Many post-transplant friends tell us that a transplant is not a cure. They encouraged Rob to simply take it easy, which is something he has trouble allowing himself to do. Rob gets antsy if he doesn't have something to do and begins to especially worry about finances. Transitioning into normal life will be challenging.

While I do not expect perfection, I believe Rob and I will now be able to communicate on a deeper level, knowing for sure that we have each other's back. We hope to find our way back to each other so that our individual and collective needs are met. But everything takes time. We have been through so much together.

We have the power to be content or restless, fulfilled or bereft, unselfish or selfish, confident or worried. As my mother always stressed, "know the difference between problems and inconveniences."

Rob received a new engine inside him, which now flushes out the old angry toxins in his body. With that comes the responsibility to take care of himself physically, mentally, and emotionally. Sure, there are things that will still make him angry, but hopefully he can keep it in better perspective.

The kids have a healthier father who will be present in their lives. And I received a husband who looks and acts younger every day. Sure, he is still fifty-six, but hopefully he will now be more spontaneous, adventurous, and amorous.

While the traditional idea of romance is often promoted, marriages are constantly tested by everyday realities of life. Each of us has our own expectations in relationships, which become conditional, whether we realize it or not. Sometimes we simply have to change our expectations during challenging times.

This experience taught us how to remain resilient during crisis and not give up. Even through the most difficult times, we have to stay in the moment, not jump too far ahead, or be stuck in the past. Planning ahead in a general sense is important, but we also need to be flexible with change and trust that everything will work out the way it is supposed to. It may not be what is expected, but hoping for the best while preparing for the worst keeps us rooted in the present.

My role, as caregiver and spouse, has been different. The caregiver responds to the patient emotionally, often feeling helpless in trying to help. We are hoping our patient has relief. Everything becomes centered around them, and we have held a lot of responsibility keeping ourselves and our family together. While I did not experience direct trauma to my body, I realize that my emotional trauma has been profound, and it will take time to heal and rediscover myself.

As transplant recipient Louis says, "Once we are that sick, the only thing we are thinking about is that illness. We don't see the emotions of other people. We don't see the suffering of others."

As transplant recipient Jerry says, "Transplant is only the beginning."

And as transplant recipient Andy says, "The caregiver's role is the hardest."

"I'm tired of chasing the dollar," Rob told a good friend recently. "I want to simplify my life, live within our means, and spend quality time with my family and friends because time is the most important commodity we have. It's all about time. My time has been extended, and I appreciate every bit of it."

We don't know what the future will hold. But we are going to live in the moment and find out.

Here's to second chances!

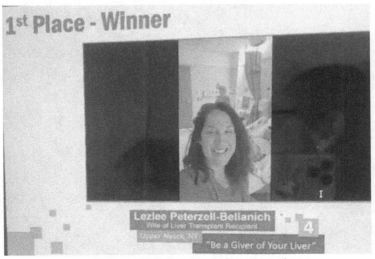

Winner of Allocare Transplant Festival

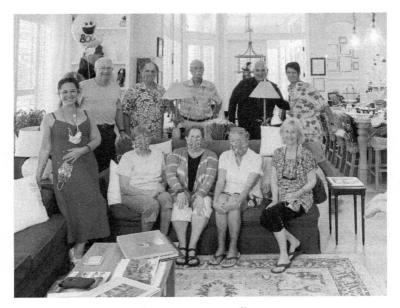

Support group goodbye

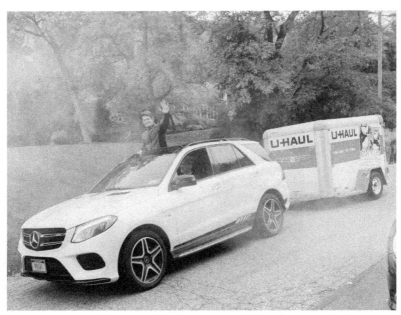

Welcome Home Parade in Nyack

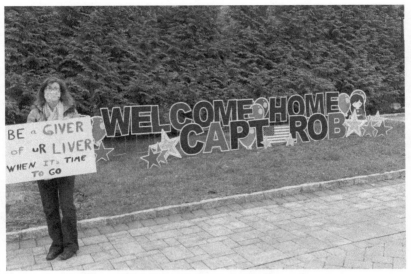

Lezlee and Rob's friend Angela holds the perfect sign

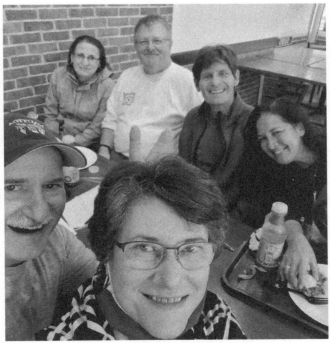

Reunion with some of the Bellanich family

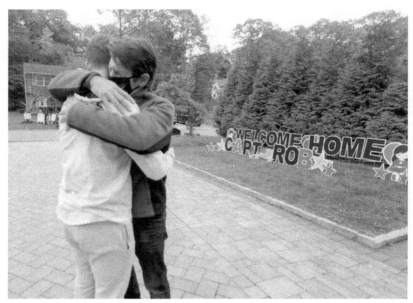

Rob reunited with River at home

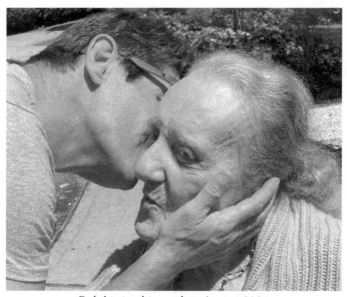

Rob kissing his mother, August 2021

Rob's Letter to His Donor Family

Tuesday, May 18, 2021

Dearest Donor Family,

It has been eight months since receiving my liver transplant on September 10, 2020. I see each day as a gift and send you my sincere gratitude for giving me a second chance at life.

My name is Rob. I am a 56-year-old male married to a wonderful wife, Lezlee, for almost 20 years. We have two children named River, age 16, and Skye, age 12. I was diagnosed with a very rare autoimmune disorder called Primary Sclerosing Cholangitis (PSC) in 2003, just two years after being married. PSC causes scarring of the bile ducts, which leads to cirrhosis of the liver. There is no cure.

I think of my donor every day. I have a part of this person inside me, now keeping me alive. My donor liver is doing very well. Before the transplant, I was jaundiced, extremely fatigued, thin from muscle-mass wasting, and so afraid. I lost my father to cirrhosis of the liver when I was 17 years old and was scared my wife and children would suffer the same fate.

Not knowing anything about the person who donated their precious organ to me is sad. I would love to know who he or she was and be able to thank the family. While I can only imagine how painful your loss is, please know that this gift has freed me from an 18-year battle with a progressive disease with no known cause that was a shadow over my life. I am forever grateful.

I hope to communicate with you soon,

Love,

Rob

Author's Notes

There are many important organ transplantation statistics. I am listing a few below but encourage readers to go to my website, www.Lezlee.com for a more extensive glossary of terms and resources.

- ✓ Deceased donors make up the majority of organ donations, yet only three in 1,000 deaths occur in a way that allows for organ donation. (American Transplant Foundation)
- ✓ One deceased donor can save up to eight lives through organ donation. (organdonor.gov)
- ✓ Ninety percent of adults in the United States support organ donation, but only sixty percent are signed up as donors. (organdonor.gov)
- ✓ A shortage of organs for transplant means that 8,000 people die each year (almost one per hour) because the organs they need are not available in time. (donatelife.net)

So far, since Rob's liver transplant, all of his blood work has proved to be perfect. His donor liver is working beautifully. He has tapered off certain medicine, and his lifelong anti-rejection medicine is being monitored and tweaked. The results of the biopsy at the four-month follow-up in early 2021 indicated no malignant cells. This was incredible news.

My petition to the United Network for Organ Sharing (UNOS) has received more than 9,500 signatures. Many of these people who were affected by PSC wrote on the public comment section of UNOS (unos.org). The Organ Procurement Transplant Network (OPTN) recently proposed an important policy change, which the National Liver Review Board approved in June 2021. It basically makes it less restrictive for doctors to request exception points on MELD scores for PSC patients. Instead of a patient having to be hospitalized twice or more in two months with sepsis, doctors can request exception points if these patients have been hospitalized twice in one year. Candidates must be admitted to the hospital with a documented blood stream infection or evidence of sepsis including hemodynamic instability requiring vasopressors.

For more information on being an organ donor, please visit www.donatelife.net.

And, if you are interested in transplantation or would like to know more, I hope you will reach out to me at author@lezlee.com and to others to ask questions, discuss, and share information through my website, www.lezlee.com. Please sign up for my email newsletter, and I look forward to hearing from you!

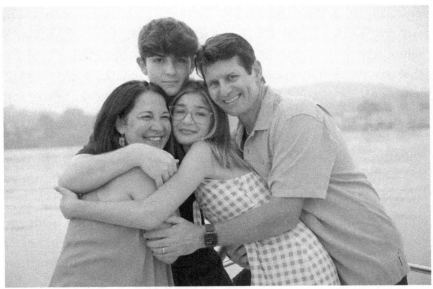

Bellanich family, July 2021

Acknowledgments

First and foremost, thank you to my husband, Captain Rob, who endured eighteen years with the autoimmune disease that affected him emotionally and psychologically before ravaging his liver. His story shaped my story, which led to the creation of this book.

River and Skye, our beloved children, are our greatest pride and joy. They were troopers throughout our entire ordeal and are becoming amazing human beings.

To our donor, whoever you are, you gave Rob the greatest gift … the gift of life. We are forever indebted. One day, we hope to meet your family.

Thank you to the entire transplant team at Mayo Clinic, especially to Rob's surgeon, Dr. Shennen Mao; hepatologists, Dr. Andrew Keaveny and Dr. Raj Satyanarayana; Tommy Mulligan, senior organ procurement coordinator, who beautifully explains the transplantation system; and Michael Womack, social worker, who leads the Second Chance Support Group. Sharing stories and supporting each other each week through this incredible medical miracle continues to be invaluable. Transplant centers across the country should have a regular support group.

Also, special thanks to the late Lisa Schaffner, former director of marketing and public relations at UNOS, for connecting me with others at the organization and helping shape my voice for PSC patients. With Lisa's recommendation, I became a UNOS Ambassador, one of the volunteer advocates working to raise awareness of organ donation and educate the public. Lisa unexpectedly passed away before this book was published. My interview with her can be read on my website.

I am so grateful to the special people in this book and others I spoke with who so openly shared their survival stories and trusted me to write them. You were there for us and continue to help others who want a second chance at life.

To my family on the Bellanich and Peterzell/Hoffman side, my amazing friends, our hard-working crew, and incredible community both in New York and newfound ones in Florida (too many to name)—thank you. We could not have done this without your love and support. Some of you we relied on to keep our business afloat, our Nyack home intact, oversee our children, comfort, and just be present in our lives.

As a first-time author, I valued the enormous input and encouragement from my author uncle, Roy Hoffman, who discussed my manuscript possibilities at length, and my aunt, Robbie Nadas, who painstakingly edited early drafts of this manuscript.

If it weren't for a woman named Cathy Schultz who works at the Book Loft on Amelia Island, Florida, and my sister-in-law, Amy, who suggested we visit there, I would not have connected with my fabulous publishers, Marie and Mark Fenn of Giro Di Mondo, and my talented editor, Emily Carmain. All the stars aligned.

Thank you to my mother in heaven, Becky Hoffman, for loving and supporting me throughout my whole life and now even in death. And to my late father, Marc Peterzell, I miss you and know you would be so proud. Thank you both for giving me my lifelong loyal sibling, Scott Peterzell, whom I love with all my heart.

Knowledge is power. Hope is vital.

About the Author

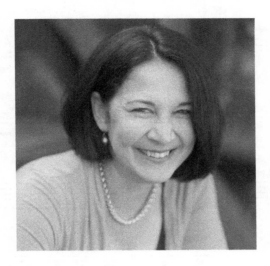

After eighteen years of marriage, the life of Lezlee Peterzell-Bellanich, singer/songwriter and business owner, took a dramatic turn. *Saved by a Stranger* is the story of her husband's harrowing quest for a liver transplant. With their two children, the Bellanich family temporarily relocated from New York to Florida during the height of the Covid pandemic. This bold additional upheaval would increase Rob's chances of receiving a deceased organ. Meeting weekly with fellow transplant patients and caregivers at Mayo Clinic's support group, the couple found solace and encouragement from these survivors' stories. Visit the author at www.lezlee.com

Be a Giver of Your Liver

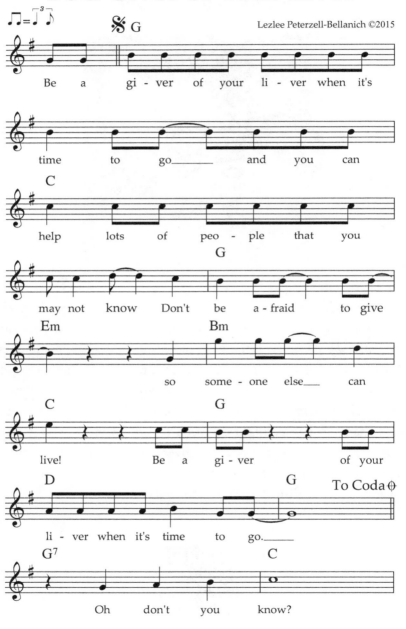

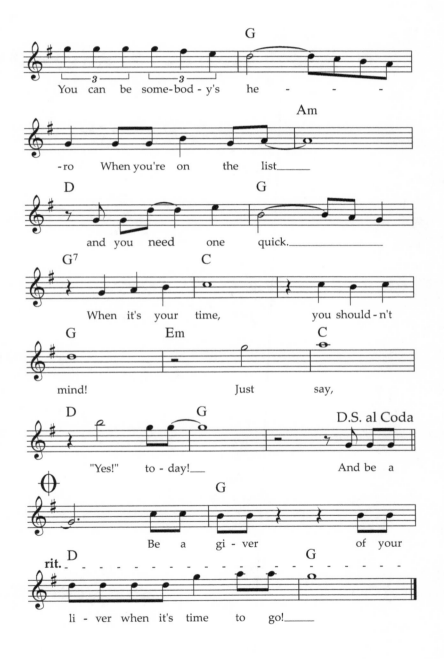

CPSIA information can be obtained
at www.ICGtesting.com
Printed in the USA
LVHW112110181021
700793LV00003B/5/J